# Slimming World

## food with
# family & friends

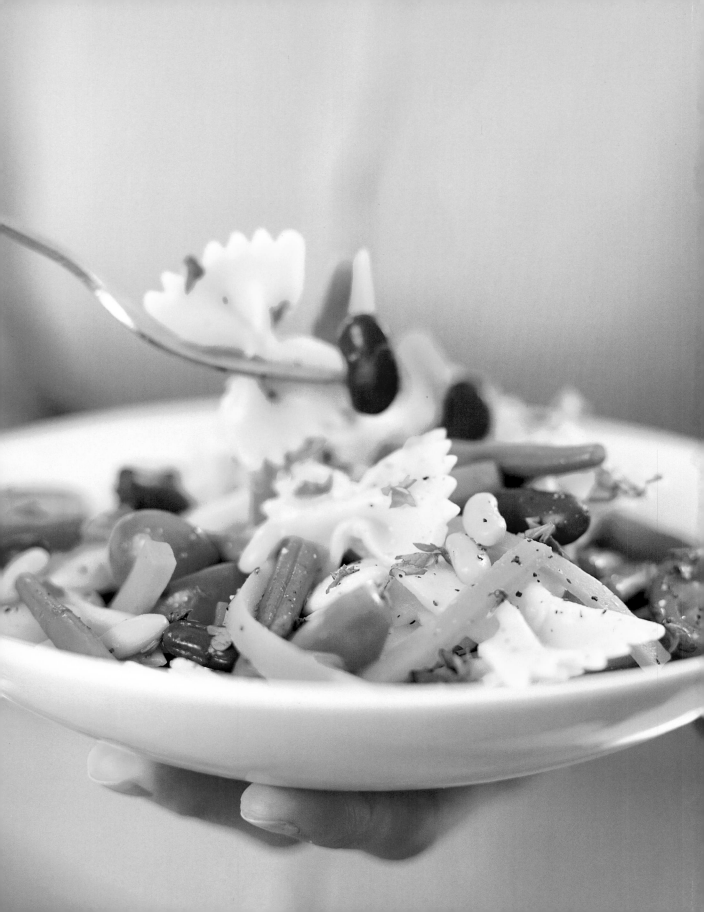

# Slimming World
## food with
# family & friends

### Great food for healthy living

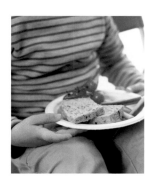 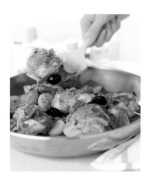 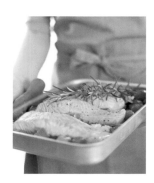

EBURY
PRESS

5  6  7  8  9  10

Published in 2004 by Ebury Press, an imprint of Ebury Publishing

A Random House Group company

The Random House Group LImited Reg. No. 954009

The Random House Group Limited supports The Forest Stewardship Council (FSC),
the leading international forest certification organisation. All our titles that are printed
on Greenpeace approved FSC certified paper carry the FSC logo.
Our paper procurement policy can be found at www.randomhouse.co.uk/environment

Addresses for companies within the Random House Group can be found at www.randomhouse.co.uk

A CIP catalogue record for this book is available from the British Library

Project editor: Emma Callery
Recipes created by Sunil Vijayakar
Design: Sue Miller

Food photography: Jon Whitaker
Food stylist: Sunil Vijayakar
Prop stylist: Antonia Gaunt

For Slimming World
Founder and Chairman: Margaret Miles-Bramwell
Managing Director: Caryl Richards
Project co-ordinator: Allison Brentnall
Text by Christine Michael

Printed and bound in China

ISBN 978  0 09 189604 1

# Slimming World

Founded in 1969 by Margaret Miles-Bramwell, Slimming World is the UK's most advanced slimming organisation. It currently manages thousands of groups across the country with over 250,000 members attending every month, and another 15,000 attending free as successful target members. Each week, around 2,000 members reach their personal target weight. Slimming World's unique approach to weight loss is an extraordinary success story.

## Cookery notes

■ Both metric and imperial measures are given for the recipes. Please follow either set of measures as they are not interchangeable.

■ All spoon measures are level: 1 tsp = 5ml spoon, 1 tbsp = 15ml spoon.

■ Ovens should be preheated to the specified temperature. Grills should also be preheated.

■ Use large eggs unless otherwise specified.

■ Note that some of the dessert recipes contain raw or lightly cooked eggs. Avoid serving these to anyone who is pregnant or in a vulnerable health group, because of the small risk of salmonella infection.

■ We'd recommend using fresh herbs for best results, unless dried herbs are suggested in the recipe.

■ For best results use freshly ground black pepper and sea salt unless otherwise specified.

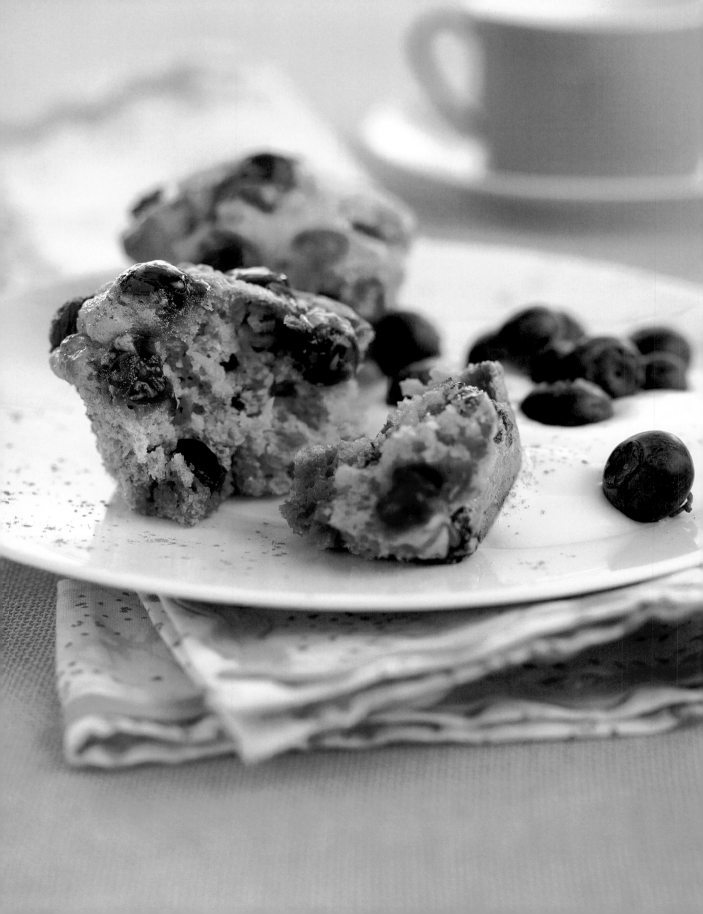

# Contents

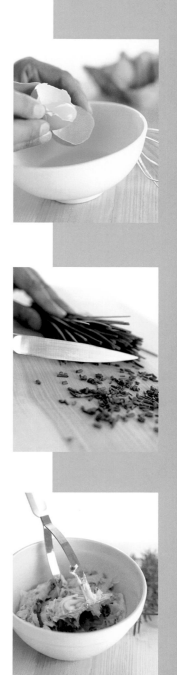

# Foreword

**Dear Reader**

As **Slimming World's** Founder and Chairman I am especially delighted to welcome you to a book called **Food with Family & Friends,** as for me it has a double meaning. Of course, this book contains a gorgeous collection of recipes that you will love to share with friends or family, in the certain and joyful knowledge that you can indeed enjoy delicious food and a good social life when you are aiming to slim or maintain your weight.

But more than this, I hope you will be inspired by this book to find out more about good food and good friends, by joining one of our warm and friendly groups. At **Slimming World** we always say that there are no strangers; only friends you haven't yet met. A **Slimming World** group is the best place to learn a little about our uniquely slimmer-friendly organisation, to experience a taste of Food Optimising and discover what it can really do for your weight-loss campaign.

As someone who knows only too well how it feels to struggle with being overweight, over 30 years ago I made it my personal life goal to do everything I could to help fellow slimmers release themselves from the diet trap and the misery it brings. For me, this meant finding a way of losing weight that was generous and enjoyable, as well as effective and healthy, and, above all, a plan that fitted into everyone's life so that they could stick to it for life, not just until they stepped off the 'diet treadmill'.

Today, I am incredibly proud that **Slimming World** is the UK's leading weight-loss organisation, with thousands of friendly groups held each week throughout the country. I am thrilled that hundreds of thousands of slimmers around the country have discovered the power of Food Optimising – the most generous, the most effective, and the most flexible weight-loss system ever.

There is nothing faddy or gimmicky about Food Optimising; it is based on sound, current nutritional thinking, so that you can be confident that you are losing weight in the safest, healthiest way that scientists recommend today. Yet it's so much more than that too. At **Slimming World** you will find an amazingly supportive network of friends who can help you through the difficulties that every slimmer faces, because they've been there themselves. And you can learn to use the immensely powerful motivational tools that we have developed over the years, based on our deep understanding of the needs and concerns of slimmers.

That is why I am so excited every time I have the opportunity to share our wonderful approach to slimming with someone who loves food and believes that means they will never be able to lose weight, or someone who has tried other diets and found them far too guilt-inducing and restrictive. Someone like you, perhaps!

If we are meeting for the first time through this book, a very warm welcome to **Slimming World.** I hope that we have given you the inspiration for many lovely, memorable gatherings of food and friends. And I hope that if you are at the point where you wish to change your life, you will join us and allow us the privilege of welcoming you to a whole new world of food, friends – and success.

**Margaret Miles-Bramwell**
**Founder and Chairman**
**Slimming World**

# Food Optimising:
# the secret ingredient

**Welcome to Slimming World's *Food with Family & Friends*, a collection of easy, delicious recipes that you'll love to share. We hope they'll inspire you to have fun and to create special occasions that you and your guests will remember for the fabulous food as well as the great time you had.**

If you're new to Slimming World, the recipes we supply may also intrigue you: what is a leading weight-loss organisation doing, producing a book about entertaining and actually **enjoying** a foody social life? After all, diet recipes are OK if you're on a diet, but you wouldn't want to inflict them on anyone else, surely? And you certainly wouldn't throw a party based on them – or would you?

Just a glance through this book will show you that the recipes in *Food with Family & Friends* are anything but typical 'diet food'. You'll find generous servings of delicious foods that are usually restricted on weight-loss diets, foods such as creamy risottos, succulent steaks, pasta bakes, luxury fish and seafood dishes, and mouth-watering desserts – with sauces, dressings and trimmings that you'd expect to find at a gourmet meal. Present your guests with a dish from *Food with Family & Friends* and they'll never believe that you could regularly enjoy so much delicious food and still lose weight. And as resident chef you may find it hard to believe yourself!

Nonetheless, it's true: you can cook from *Food with Family & Friends* every single day and still be confident that you will be following a healthy, effective weight-loss plan. That's because these recipes have a 'secret ingredient': they've all been devised using Slimming World's unique and sophisticated way of eating that helps you to lose weight without ever needing to go hungry, and without depriving yourself (or your friends) of the foods you enjoy.

**Hundreds of thousands of successful slimmers have already discovered this special secret**, by attending one of the 5,500 warm and friendly Slimming World groups held across the country every week. They have found Food Optimising. And they have discovered that with Food Optimising you really can:

- **Eat to slim** instead of starving yourself to slim.
- Feel **relaxed**, **free** and **in control** around food.
- Slim while **enjoying** normal, everyday meals with family and friends.
- Be **confident** that you are **eating healthily** while achieving your weight-loss goal.

■ **Lose weight** while **eating** a vast range of foods you enjoy in **unlimited** amounts.

■ Satisfy your appetite so that you need **never go hungry**.

■ Enjoy your favourite treats every day if **you choose**.

■ **Eat, live life and enjoy food in a new way – for life**.

Having chosen this book, you may well be one of the millions of people who'd love to lose weight but believe whole-heartedly that life is for living. Sharing a meal and a laugh with friends and family is one of life's great pleasures, but many weight-loss methods are so restrictive or inflexible that they can seem impossible to combine with a normal social life. If you have tried diets like this before, it's no wonder they didn't work for you.

Slimming World understands, better than any other weight-loss organisation, that a successful way of losing weight and keeping it off has to fit in with YOUR lifestyle, not the other way round. That's because our philosophy is based on a deep understanding of how people with a weight problem feel, coupled with a passionate desire to help them achieve their goals. We have over 30 years of experience helping people reach the weight they want to be and we start from where you are; we love food, friends and having fun every bit as much as you do, and we're not prepared to give up all of those things to lose weight any more than you are.

**We love food, friends and having fun every bit as much as you do, and we're not prepared to give up all of those things to lose weight any more than you are.**

Because it's based on the real needs and wants of slimmers, Food Optimising offers a very different approach to weight loss from diets you may have tried or read about before. Since it was launched over 30 years ago, Food Optimising has been refined and developed in line with current nutritional thinking. You can be confident that

## Food Optimising is based on:

■ Foods that fill you so well, you can **eat as much** of them as you like.

■ Foods that typically all diets **ban**.

■ Foods that **speed** your weight loss.

■ Foods that **boost** vitamins and minerals, calcium and fibre.

when you are Food Optimising you are eating in a way that is known to be healthy for people who wish to lose weight today. And the principles and the passion that made Food Optimising so revolutionary back then are even stronger today. **Food Optimising is still the most generous, most flexible, most satisfying and most slimmer-friendly way of losing weight and maintaining your healthy weight that you will find – anywhere!**

## The freedom of Food Optimising

So many claims are made for weight-loss 'miracles' and celebrity-endorsed 'wonder-diets' that it would be understandable if you felt sceptical about what the Slimming World approach has to offer. So right from the start, let's be clear that there is nothing faddy or 'weird' about Food Optimising.

It is based on the scientific fact, agreed by all the experts, that to lose weight you have to alter your 'energy balance'. In other words, that you have to take in fewer calories (energy units) than you expend, so that your body gradually uses up the energy it has stored in the form of fat.

With traditional weight-loss diets, slimmers are encouraged to alter their energy balance by monitoring their calorie intake, weighing and measuring everything they eat, and by cutting down or cutting out high-calorie foods.

At Slimming World we have always known that a slimmer wants plenty of gorgeous food – and having far too little of it is not a course of action that could last long. Your body would crave the comfort of a really satisfying meal and your mind would be tormented by the food you were being denied.

**Our unique approach to slimming is based on a revolutionary concept – that of 'Free Foods' – foods that you can eat without restriction, any time, anywhere, whenever you need to eat.**

That's not the way to get slim and stay slim. Restricting intake too much results in the loss of more lean tissue (such as muscle) from our bodies as well as body fat. Loss of lean tissue has unfavourable effects on our metabolic rate: the more we lose, the more our metabolic rate will fall. This is why experts recommend gradual weight loss on a sensible calorie intake – and not severely calorie-restricted (crash) diets. So, like many other strokes of genius, Food Optimising takes the accepted wisdom and stands it on its head: it encourages you to eat Free Foods. Our unique approach to slimming is based on a revolutionary concept – that of 'Free Foods' – foods that you can eat without restriction, any time, anywhere, whenever you need to eat.

These **Free Foods** aren't just typical diet staples such as lettuce leaves and low-fat cottage cheese. We're talking about choices such as pasta, rice, potatoes, lean meat, fish, poultry, and all the fresh fruit and vegetables you can eat, without having to weigh or measure a single spoonful.

Fancy a big plateful of vegetable curry with unlimited rice, or a pile of pasta with a spicy tomato sauce? How about a monster jacket potato with a tin of baked beans? Then again, you might like a proper roast dinner with plenty of lean meat and loads of vegetables. Or a big, fluffy omelette stuffed with ham. Or a meaty tuna steak with a heap of ratatouille. All of these meals – and there are hundreds more besides — can be eaten freely; that is as **Free Foods**, when you're Food Optimising, depending on whether you choose a Green day or Original day. More about that later on pages 19–20.

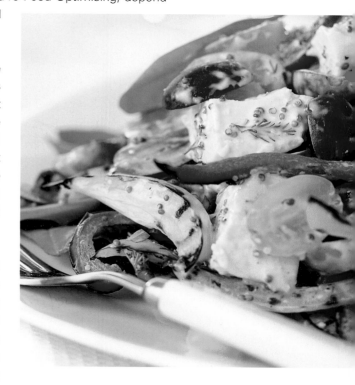

If you were sceptical before, you might think we've gone mad by encouraging slimmers to eat as much as they like! If so, you're not alone; initially, to many diet experts, Slimming World's **Free Foods** seem quite outrageous. Even some of our members are doubtful at first. They return to their group, after their first week of Food Optimising, having determined to 'prove us wrong' by eating as much **Free Food** as they can, only to find that they've lost weight – and lots of it.

The concept of **Free Foods** runs against conventional thinking in two ways. First, if eating too much has made you overweight in the first place, how can you eat as much as you like and hope to lose weight? And second, how can you ensure that you are altering your energy balance (i.e. reducing your overall energy intake) when you aren't weighing and measuring everything you eat?

The answer to the first question lies in Slimming World's deep understanding of slimmers and a desire to free them from the guilt and the self-blame that many restrictive diet systems impose. The fact is that there are many slimmers who live their lives in fear of consuming 'forbidden foods' and 'eating too much'. They are judged, criticised and 'told off' for eating so much. They are often made to feel like naughty children who should be told what to do, what to eat and when to eat it. It's hardly surprising if, no matter how much we want to lose weight, we rebel when we're treated in this way.

If you've ever experienced a weight-loss 'lecture' from a poker-faced person who looks as though they've never had a weight problem, you'll know it's no laughing matter. Trying to follow eating plans that leave you feeling deprived, hungry or worthless (or, worse still, all three), often results in a destructive pattern of being 'on a diet', followed by going 'off the diet' to eat normally again when the urge becomes overwhelming. This can lead to thinking about certain foods as 'good' or 'bad' and thinking about yourself as 'good' or 'bad', depending on what foods you are eating. Instead of blaming the diet for failing you, you blame yourself for failing, so your motivation sinks even lower and you have even less chance of achieving your goal.

**When you are freed from the fear of hunger, the urge to overeat disappears. Control comes from choice power, not cast-iron willpower.**

At Slimming World we firmly believe that our members are wonderful, warm, competent people who are more than capable of managing their lives and their weight. Experience has shown us that offering slimmers unrestricted access to a wide range of foods doesn't mean that they will 'go overboard'. In practice, we find that if you can have **Free Foods** in quantity, you don't actually eat them in quantity. **There is no need to deny yourself, or eat guiltily. When you are freed from the fear of hunger, the urge to overeat disappears**, and behaviour around food becomes much more rational. Decisions become real, not enforced; control comes from choice power, not cast-iron willpower.

So when we say you can eat as much as you like of a wide variety of **Free Foods** we mean exactly that … as much as you like! This is the liberation that persuades many people that Food Optimising will work for them, even if they have tried and failed at every other weight-loss system you can think of. It brings a freedom and an enlightenment to your weight-loss journey that you previously thought impossible.

## The heart of Food Optimising

Do you hate the very word calorie? Most of us have had a run-in with calorie-counting at some point during our search for a slimmer shape. In fact, calorie-counting is possibly the most hated way to lose weight. Yet all experts agree that you have to lower your calorie intake in order to lose weight. But how can you achieve this and not run out of things to eat by mid-afternoon?

**Food Optimising is the only eating plan that deals with the practical and the psychological needs of slimmers.**

This leads us to the heart of Food Optimising: the **only** eating plan that deals with the practical and the psychological needs of slimmers, and that takes into account up-to-the-minute scientific thinking on the relationship between appetite, overeating and dieting, coupled with an understanding of why people behave around food as they do.

**Food Optimising is based on the principle that being able to satisfy your appetite on foods you love is the key to losing weight successfully and, just as importantly, to maintaining a healthy weight for life.**

When you follow Food Optimising, you will be eating more of the foods that satisfy your appetite most effectively. You will automatically be making healthier food choices, which naturally limit your overall calorie intake without counting a single calorie, and you will feel less need for high-sugar, high-fat snacks that pile on the calories (and the pounds) while providing no nutritional benefit.

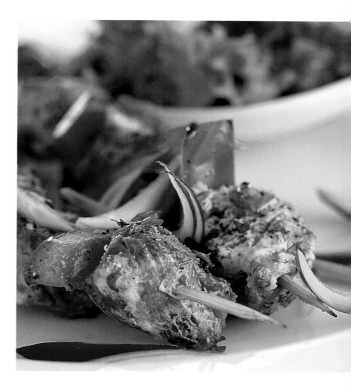

Our body controls our appetite by sending out different signals at various points as we digest our food, from chewing right through to absorption of the nutrients we've consumed. Some signals tell us to stop wanting more food when our body doesn't need any more (that's called satiation) and other signals prevent us from wanting to eat again until our body requires

**You will automatically be making healthier food choices, which naturally limit your overall calorie intake without counting a single calorie.**

more energy (known as satiety). Food Optimising takes all this into account. Some years ago, Slimming World sponsored research into whether certain types of food were better at prompting satiation and satiety signals than others. The results showed that of the major food groups, protein headed the list, followed by carbohydrates. Trailing well behind was fat.

Foods rich in protein (for example, lean meat and fish) and those rich in carbohydrates (such as pasta and potatoes) are some of the most important in triggering these signals of satiation and satiety. These are the foods that form the basis of Slimming World's revolutionary **Free Foods** list.

When you are Food Optimising you are positively encouraged to eat plenty of foods in these food groups to satisfy your appetite and keep you feeling fuller for longer.

The other big advantage of these major food groups for slimmers is that many foods that are rich in protein and carbohydrates are low in energy density. Energy density describes the amount of calories within (or provided by) a certain weight of food. It is the equivalent of calories per gram. Foods that are low in energy density, such as fruit and vegetables, lean meat, fish and poultry, and rice, pasta and potatoes, take time to eat. They are bulky, fill you up and make it more difficult to consume a lot of calories and so are good news for slimmers. On the other hand, foods that are high in energy density, such as fats, oil and sugar, have a lot of calories packed into a small volume; they can be eaten quickly and can lead to a high calorie intake within a short time. By choosing foods with low energy density – **Free Foods** – you can still eat the same amount of food (or more) and feel satisfied, yet you will be automatically reducing your calorie intake.

# You choose

Food Optimising offers you **another clever way** to help you limit your overall energy intake in an easy, stress-free, enjoyable way, by asking you **to choose** between two types of daily menu: **Green** and **Original**.

■ On a **Green day**, your plate will be full of carbohydrate-rich foods such as **unlimited potatoes, pasta or rice**, with loads of green vegetables and a **measured** amount of **lean meat or fish**.
■ On an **Original day**, your plate will be piled high with protein-rich foods such as **unlimited lean meat or fish**, loads of green vegetables once again, and a **measured** portion of **pasta, rice or potatoes**.

Some people like to stick to **Green days or Original days**; others have a mixture of **Green and Original days**. You're in control; you choose.

You can see from the way we describe the Green and Original choices that Food Optimising is quite unlike food combining, where protein-rich and carbohydrate-rich foods are not allowed to be eaten together in the same meal. With Food Optimising you simply have smaller portions of some foods knowing that other, really filling and great-tasting, foods are on hand all day long.

■ On a **Green day**, for example, you could choose a measured serving of cooked chicken tossed into a huge, tasty vegetable stir-fry with unlimited spicy noodles.
■ Or on an **Original day** you could have a succulent salmon steak in a low-fat creamy sauce, with a measured serving of new potatoes and lots of freshly cooked green vegetables.

## Helping you to choose

■ To help you make your choices for Green and Original days we have colour-coded the recipes in this book to indicate which recipes are lower in Syns on each choice: **green for Green days** and **blue for Original days**.

■ If a recipe is **Free** on both Green and Original days, we have coloured it **lilac**.

■ If a recipe has the **same number of Syns** on Green and Original, we have coloured it **green** *and* **blue**.

Food Optimising is not about separating different types of nutrients, but about allowing you to choose the proportions of different types of food you prefer. It allows you to fill up on the foods you choose to satisfy your taste buds and your appetite on that particular day and then add other foods for balance without having to worry about counting or measuring. If you want to fill up on potatoes, pasta and rice (which contain lots of satiating complex carbohydrates) or perhaps beans, peas and lentils (which contain complex carbohydrates and are a good source of protein, too) then opt for the **Green choice**, and you can do so freely. If on some days you feel like satisfying your appetite with lean meat, poultry or fish (rich in protein), then you can choose an **Original day**. You can always add fruit and green vegetables (which contain some carbohydrate) to any meal quite freely on both Green and Original days. Some non-meat proteins, such as Quorn and tofu, are **Free Foods** on **Green** and **Original days**, and eggs (high in protein) are also **Free Foods** on both **Green** and **Original days**.

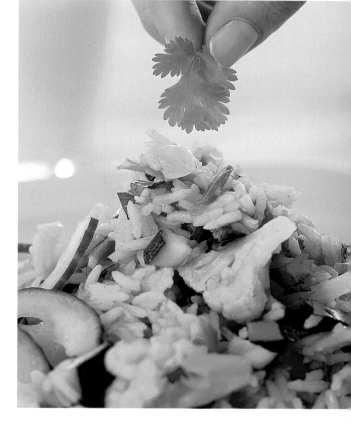

This ability to **mix and match** your meals according to your appetite and your lifestyle makes Food Optimising so flexible that it really is a way of managing your weight and eating **healthily for life**. That's the great part – Food Optimising is designed to work forever. It's **long-term healthy eating**, it's your eating lifestyle **for the twenty-first century**.

**Your lifestyle, your choice:** with Food Optimising we

## Eat, enjoy and lose weight

■ Food Optimising **doesn't entail strict rules**, an in-depth knowledge of nutrition, or taking time to calculate what's in your food.

■ The principles of Food Optimising take care of all that for you, so all you have to do is **eat, enjoy, and lose weight**.

■ Once you have made Food Optimising a habit, you will find that it becomes second nature, fitting **easily** and **comfortably** into your lifestyle.

don't tell you what to eat at every meal; **you are in control** of what you eat and when you eat it. Slimming World members soon learn how to manage the huge range of choices they have. If you join us, you'll find you'll be planning your own daily and weekly menus based on the foods you enjoy eating, and which will keep your appetite **satisfied all day**.

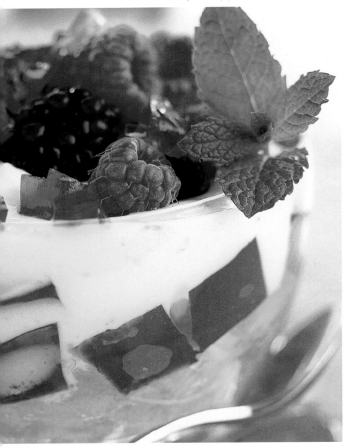

Eating in this way is so flexible and free-ing. If you associate 'dieting' with having to cook separate meals for yourself, and refusing invitations to eat out, you will find that **Food Optimising** is a **glorious liberation** from all that self-denial.

Because Food Optimising recipes are based on the very best principles of nutrition, they can be used even if you don't want to lose weight. Your family and friends will enjoy them too. Eating in this way helps you to keep a stable weight through life. Most of us worry that we will put on weight as we get older – but that's no longer inevitable. In fact, with Food Optimising, you're in the driving seat – for good!

Welcome to the **most advanced** weight-loss system you've ever found.

**Welcome to Food Optimising.**

# Step by step to Food Optimising

**In the previous section we looked at some of the scientific principles behind Food Optimising and how what might seem to be a 'miraculous' weight loss system is actually based on sound nutrition and advanced behavioural science.**

However, the great news is that you don't need to be a nutrition expert to Food Optimise successfully: you can get going at once just by following a few straightforward guidelines.

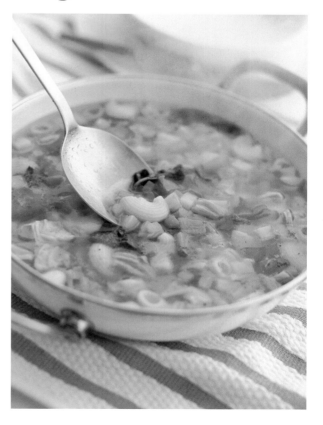

### Step 1: Go for Free Foods

You've already found that each day we ask you to **make a choice** to have a **Green day** or an **Original day** and to stick to that choice all day. Whichever day you choose, you will find there is a huge list of **Free Foods** for you to enjoy. On page 220 we give you some examples of **Free Foods** for both **Green** and **Original days**.

As we have seen, what all these **Free Foods** have in common is that they are **low in energy density** and **high in appetite satisfaction**. And because there are so many of them and you can prepare them into such delicious meals, you could quite easily lose weight by eating **Free Foods** all day, without having to weigh, measure or worry about what you're eating at all. That sounds amazing in itself, but then you get to eat some more!

### Step 2: Eat a healthy balance

As well as all the **Free Foods,** every day we ask you to choose measured portions of **Healthy Extras**, more long lists of foods that boost your fibre, vitamins and minerals, especially calcium, which is vital for good health and, according to the latest research, may play an important part in helping the body to metabolise fat.

**Healthy Extras** can include wholemeal bread, high-fibre breakfast cereals, soups

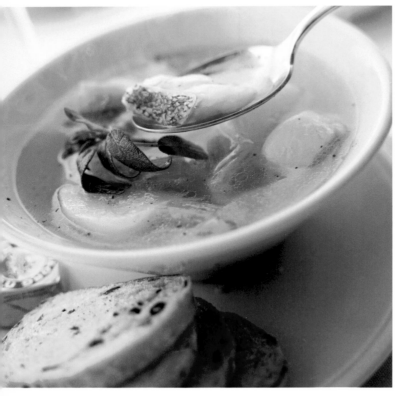

and dairy products.

**On Green days,** the **Healthy Extras** list includes:

■ Lean meat ■ Fish ■ Poultry.

**On Original days**, you could also choose:

■ Potatoes ■ Pasta ■ Pulses.

**A few words about fibre**

Getting **enough fibre** is important in any healthy diet, whether you are trying to lose weight or not. Generally in the UK, we don't eat enough fibre, which can increase our risk of developing conditions ranging from constipation to much more serious illnesses such as cancer of the colon and even heart disease (as dietary fibre helps to reduce cholesterol).

The good news here is that **Food Optimising** makes the most of **fibre-rich foods**, for the least amount of calories. Fruit and vegetables, for instance, are not only rich in fibre and a powerful protection against many diseases, they're also low in energy density, so they are **Free Foods** when you are Food Optimising. Official healthy-eating guidelines say you should aim for five portions of fruit and veg every day. We say eat at least that and as much as you can find room for! You will also find that Food Optimising encourages you to choose high-fibre foods such as wholemeal bread, wholemeal pasta and high-fibre breakfast cereals, and to add to the fibre content of meals by including beans or lentils in stews, for instance. This is partly because **high-fibre foods** are more **filling, lower in energy density** and they're also **great** for your general health.

When you start Food Optimising you may find that you are eating more fibre-rich foods than you were before. If you know your current diet is low in fibre, we advise you to increase your fibre intake relatively slowly and to drink plenty of water; this is important for good health generally but especially for helping your body process fibre-rich foods.

**On Green days,** Free Foods high in fibre include:

■ Baked beans ■ Chickpeas ■ Lentils ■ Peas ■ Quorn ■ Red kidney beans ■ Soya beans

**On Original days,** high fibre Free Foods include:
■ Artichokes ■ Broccoli ■ Brussels sprouts ■ French beans ■ Quorn ■ Runner beans.

And there's more!

**Step 3: Allow yourself to Syn a little**
Eating lots of foods that are high in energy density makes it difficult to lose weight successfully. So we recommend that Slimming World members **automatically** limit the amount of **highly energy-dense** foods they eat by allowing themselves an agreed number of Syns each day. We don't tell you how many Syns to have each day, it's your decision.

Some days, with all the delicious **Free Food** you've enjoyed, you'll be happy with as few as 5 Syns (equivalent to a glass of wine). On others, you'll need a more generous amount. For most people, between 10 and 15 Syns a day is enough to keep the pounds rolling off, while still allowing a treat every single day they are 'on a diet'! For a list of the foods people most often take as Syns, see page 221.

Every now and then, though, we all like to feel that we can 'let ourselves go' and enjoy a big night out or a special occasion. With most weight-loss systems, this is impossible; either you decide to break your diet and resign yourself to another failed attempt at slimming, or you allow yourself a chicken drumstick and a lettuce leaf from the buffet and pretend you're enjoying yourself! Not so when you're Food Optimising: **stay flexible**.

## Keep on counting

■ Count Syns **carefully** and be **realistic**.

■ If you are going to a wedding, a party or some other event and you know it will be hard to stay with a low Syn allowance for the day, estimate how many Syns you actually need. If it's 50, then accept it. Aim to **use** your 50 Syns and **enjoy them**.

■ Next day, **get back to your normal, lower allowance**.

■ It works. It works because you **stay aware** and you **stay in control**. All too often slimmers feel so guilty after eating 'too much' that they give up their healthy-eating goals altogether thinking, 'I've blown it, I just can't do it.' And they stop counting altogether for that day, that week, that month.

■ Fifty Syns can be an **awful lot less damaging** than what happens when you stop counting altogether.

As long as you're **aware** of how many Syns you're consuming (keeping a log of your daily Syn count is a good way to do this), and you stay within your **chosen upper limit** for the day, you will continue to **lose weight**. If you're having a bad day at work, you might decide you'd like 20 Syns at lunch to see you through until it's time to go home. You might decide to keep your regular night out and enjoy 50 Syns every Friday. On a very special occasion, such as a wedding, you might accept that it will even be a 100-Syn day! Agree it with yourself in advance, keep on counting and enjoy every one of those Syns on the day. The next day, return to your normal chosen allowance, knowing that you haven't ruined all your hard work and you don't need to starve yourself to make up for it.

Slimmers who are used to restrictive weight-loss methods find the idea of Slimming World's **'Flexible Syns'** completely mind-blowing, and they are sometimes scared to try it! But the secret of its success is brilliantly simple; it's based on Slimming World's understanding that although 50 or even 100 Syns sounds like an awful lot, it's undoubtedly fewer than if you'd stopped counting altogether, and certainly **less damaging** than if you'd felt you had 'really blown it' and convinced yourself there was no point in even trying again. With Food Optimising, the great thing is that while Syns are fun and important in their own way, you don't have to focus on them to lose weight successfully and enjoyably. **The vast majority of the food you will eat each day is Free Food – lots and lots of delicious, healthy and satisfying foods that will fill you up and help you slim.**

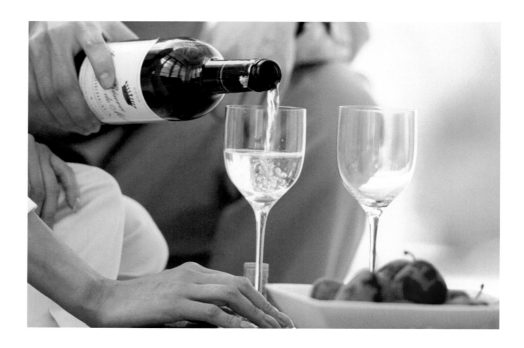

# A healthy rate of weight loss

Many new members ask **how much weight** they 'should be' losing each week at Slimming World, and again this is something that is **unique** to you. Some people lose weight every single week until they reach their target, while others prefer to take the 'scenic route'! If it works for you, it's fine by us.

Generally, we encourage a **healthy rate** of weight loss, averaging 500g–1kg (1–2lb) a week. This is a practical, **achievable** goal for most people and it encourages **realistic** expectations. Of course, everyone is different and people will lose weight at different rates influenced by a number of factors such as genetics, how much weight they have to lose, and how active they are. When people have quite a lot of weight to lose, it's not unusual to see quite large initial losses of 3–4.5kg (7–10lb) in the first week and more than 500g–1kg (1–2lb) in the following few weeks, which is partly due to the loss of water. We find, however, that for most of our members, weight loss settles to an average 500g–1kg (1–2lb) a week over time.

Top medical advisors have confirmed to us that if people are **Food Optimising** properly, a rapid weight loss isn't a problem. As long as slimmers are **eating plenty** of food, having a **balanced diet** and **exercising** to help maintain lean muscle tissue, a weight loss of more than 500g–1kg (1–2lb) a week over several weeks or even months can still be **perfectly healthy**. This is very different from crash-dieting, which just isn't possible when you're following the most generous weight-loss plan ever: **Slimming World** members regularly **enjoy** 1500–1800 calories a day.

**Learning which foods you can eat freely, and which foods you need to keep an eye on and count is a great way of learning how to eat healthily for life.** This enlightening mix of control and free-wheeling is so different and so liberating. Focusing on **Free Foods**, the kindest foods for your **well-being**, your **happiness** and your **waistline**, is so very positive.

# Body Magic

Medical experts agree that, as well as following a healthy eating plan such as Food Optimising, the best way to lose weight and to keep it off is to **become more active**. Exercising is the other key way in which we can alter our energy balance, by increasing the amount of energy we expend while we are also reducing the amount of energy we consume. However, just as restrictive diets and faddy eating regimes are counter-productive in slimming, an over-strict approach to exercising can be unhelpful too. There may be all sorts of reasons why we can't, or don't want to, take formal exercise such as sessions in the gym or going to an aerobics class. And the latest scientific evidence suggests that we don't have to go flat-out with intensive exercise in order to reap the **health benefits** of getting fitter. **Moderate, everyday activity**, such as walking briskly for 30 minutes, can be just as **effective** in helping us feel better, have more energy, and prevent some of the health problems people face when they have inactive lifestyles, such as increased risk of heart disease, stroke, diabetes and osteoporosis.

**We recognise that taking the decision to become more active needs just as much support as deciding to change your eating habits.**

At Slimming World we recognise that taking the decision to become more active needs just as much support as deciding to change your eating habits, and for that reason we've developed a powerful new tool – **Body Magic. Body Magic** has nothing to do with workout sessions in your Slimming World group or having to turn up in Lycra (unless you want to, of course!). Its aim is to **help you discover** ways in which you can **become more active** in daily life, and to **reward** and **encourage** you every step of the way.

Just as you choose what to eat when you Food Optimise, and when you would like to eat it, with **Body Magic** you **choose** when and how you would like to be more active: there are no set exercises or training schedules to follow. Whether you are an occasional exerciser who would like to make it a habit, or if you have limited mobility and find it a challenge to walk to the corner shop, Body Magic will encourage you to make progress.

Each week **you decide** how you are going to be **more active** (for example, get off the bus a stop earlier and walk, or go for a bike ride). You'll then be invited to note down your activities in your own personal FIT log (which stands for Frequency, Intensity, and Time spent). As you **build up** to the **ideal of 30 minutes of moderate activity on five days of the week**, your Consultant and fellow members will give you loads of **praise** and **support** as you share your **achievements** with your group. Your aim is to make **regular activity** a permanent part of your **lifestyle**, so that it becomes as natural as cleaning your teeth. Once you have managed this, you will have reached Slimming World's **Platinum Standard** and can look forward to enjoying the benefits of a **Body Magic lifestyle** for as long as you keep up your new level of activity.

**The Body Magic** programme fits perfectly into everything Slimming World has to offer because one of the **great benefits** of regular activity is that it **boosts** our mood and our **self-esteem**. It helps to reinforce that sense of purpose and of being the best we can be, and this is what makes our groups so powerful.

# The magic of Slimming World

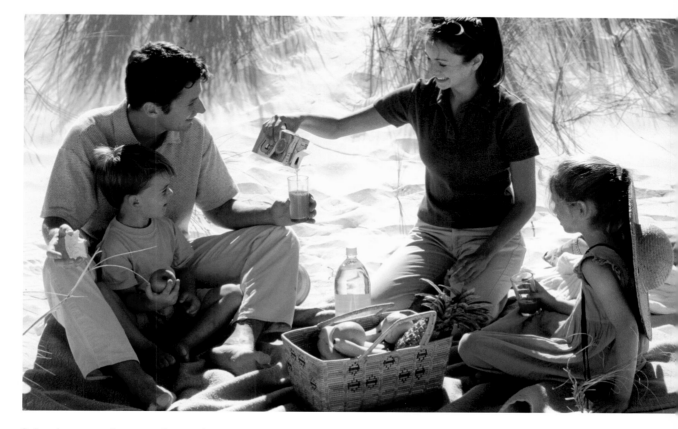

Scientists may disagree about what causes people to gain weight, but they all agree (as we saw earlier) that the key to successful weight loss is to alter the energy balance so that we expend more energy (calories) than we take in. Or to put it brutally simply: to lose weight you have to eat less and become more active.

Many weight-loss systems are based on the belief that slimmers do not actually know this information, and that all they need is to hear it repeatedly and loudly (a bit like someone who can't speak a foreign language trying to make himself understood by shouting in English). Restrictive, faddy diets, gruelling exercise regimes and systems that make slimmers feel worthless if they 'fail' all stem from this belief.

At **Slimming World**, we start from a completely opposite viewpoint. We **credit** slimmers with the intelligence to realise that they **know** they need to make **lifestyle changes** in order to lose weight and we have **faith** in their **genuine desire** to do so. We also **empathise** deeply with all the reasons why making those changes on your

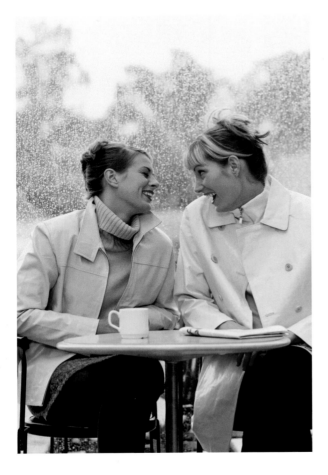

own can seem so difficult and daunting. We understand that if you have spent your life feeling ignored, discounted and disrespected because of your size, the last thing you want from a weight-loss system is to be made to feel worse.

One of the great things about joining a **Slimming World** group is that you'll find that whatever problem you face in losing weight, you are **not alone**! You'll spend time each week listening to how **fellow members** tackle the obstacles that get in the way of weight loss **success**, and you'll **learn** from each other, not from a lecturer or a textbook. It can be immensely **empowering** to find out how someone else coped with a situation such as a big night out, an urge to comfort eat, or a week when the TV beckoned more than the gym, so that you leave feeling 'I can do that!'. And one of the biggest surprises new members find at Slimming World is that they can expect **praise and support** even when – especially when — things are not going well. Every time you have had a difficult week and come back anyway (knowing how much easier it is to stay away and come back next week), your fellow members know that you are showing **courage** and **commitment**, and they applaud you for it. It's wonderful to feel the **power** and the **warmth** of that support shining on you, showing you the way forward. If your motivation is flagging, you'll leave the group feeling valued and restored, ready to start again. And if you arrived feeling positive and motivated, you will leave on an **absolute high** that's **more delicious** than any food.

We call this unique support system **Image Therapy** (**Image** stands for **I**ndividual **M**otivation **a**nd **G**roup **E**xperience) and of everything we do at Slimming World, it is probably the element we're proudest of. That's because it's based on over 30 years of **deep understanding** and of helping people to see that they have unique and wonderful qualities.

The aim of everything that happens in our groups is to increase your awareness as a member that you are worth far more than your weight, and to challenge the damaging perception that if you are overweight, there is something wrong with you. Our mission, in part, is to help you see that you are **able, imaginative, competent,**

**funny, sexy**, and more than equipped to **control** your life and your weight. **Slimming World** knows that **you have it within yourself** to make the changes you want to in your life.

**Food Optimising, Image Therapy and Body Magic are just three of the powerful tools that can help you do this. But the most empowering thought of all is that you are in control.**

## YOU decide

We all know that we have to make decisions every day. Some are big, conscious decisions, like what colour to paint the bathroom walls. Others slip by almost unnoticed, but although they seem insignificant, they can change our lives. For example, when someone last criticised you, did you agree with her inwardly instead of challenging her? Or when someone paid you a compliment, did your mind instantly dismiss it as worthless instead of acknowledging it with pleasure? Why did you decide to react that way – and what effect did your decisions have on your self-esteem?

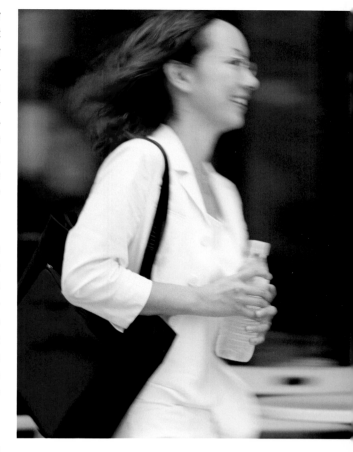

At Slimming World, we know how vital it is to be aware of the effects of the decisions we make – even the small, apparently insignificant ones, which can have such devastating results. Many weight-management systems remove your decision-making powers by telling you what to eat and when to eat it. That's a bit like learning a foreign language in phrases on an audio tape; it's fine as long as you repeat what you've learned, but what happens when you're on holiday and you have to start making real conversation?

So when you join **Slimming World** we put **you in charge** of all the **decisions** – starting with the amount of weight you would like to lose. Your **Personal Achievement Target** (PAT) is just that: it's up to **you** to **decide** the point at which you feel you would like to **celebrate your success**. Of course, if you feel, once you've got there, that you would like to set a new, lower PAT, that's fine too. Setting your own weight-loss targets puts **you** totally **in control** of the

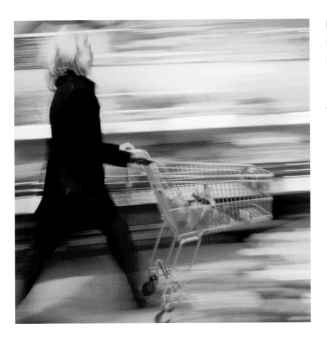

process. It also takes away that awful negative feeling that you have 'failed' if you are just a few pounds short of a target that's been set for you, no matter how much weight you may have already lost.

There is one **weight-loss** target we like **everyone** to be aware of, and that's when you've lost 10 per cent of your starting weight – for example, if you've slimmed from 20st to 18st. This is a reason to celebrate because medical evidence suggests that if you are very overweight, **losing just 10 per cent** of your excess weight brings substantial **health benefits** if you maintain that loss for ten weeks or more. Losing 10 per cent of your body weight is an achievement to be proud of and we **celebrate** this at Slimming World by making you a member of our **'Club 10'** scheme, with a further reward if you maintain your loss or go on to lose more in the next ten weeks (as many, many Club 10 members do).

**As you become aware of the decisions you are making every day, it becomes easier to take credit for the good ones, and responsibility for the less successful ones.**

Simply making a decision can be **empowering** in itself. Suppose, for instance, that you decide to join a Slimming World group that is taking place in a few days' time. For the rest of that week you might choose to eat more healthily in preparation – or you might decide to do exactly the opposite. Either way, the decision you have made to join the group will affect your behaviour, before you even go along on the day itself.

If you join **Slimming World,** you will **learn** a lot more about how **you** make decisions, and the consequences of what you decide. Each week you will be asked how much weight you would like to lose in the week to come, and if you will have any difficult choices to make, such as what to eat at a party. It's not about giving the 'right answers' and making the right decisions; it's more a question of **being aware** of the choices that will help **you achieve** your **weight-loss goal** directly, and those that will lead you to take a more leisurely journey.

**As you become aware of the decisions you are making every day, it becomes easier to take credit for the good ones, and responsibility for the ones that turn out to be less successful.**

In this introduction to our latest recipe collection, *Food for Family & Friends*, we can only give you a brief outline of what makes **Food Optimising** and **Slimming World** so successful. If you join us at Slimming World, you will find out so much more about how to make **Food Optimising** and **Body Magic** part of your lifestyle, and you will also have the invaluable **support** and **encouragement** of your Consultant and fellow members.

We're sure that if you do **join us**, you'll be so **thrilled with the results** that you'll want to tell **the world** about **Slimming World**! But even if we don't have the pleasure of meeting you in person, please don't keep the secret of these great recipes to yourself. Next time you are serving one of these meals to a friend and they ask where the recipe came from, show them this book. You never know, you could soon be receiving a thank-you note for having given them a gift that's far more valuable than a delicious meal.

**We're sure that if you do join Slimming World, you'll be so thrilled with the results that you'll want to tell the world.**

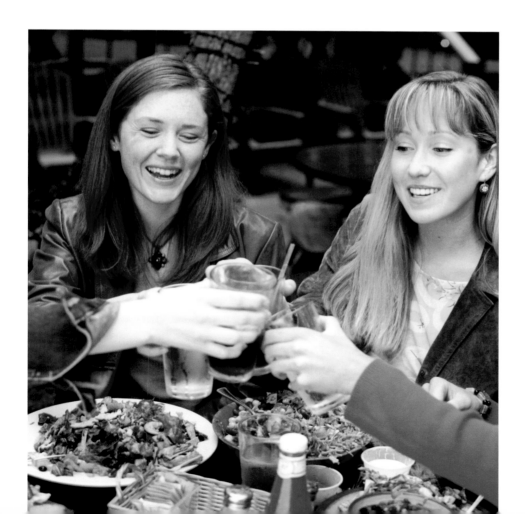

# Food Optimising menus

**Take a week or two to follow our tasty selection of mouth-watering menus and you'll be able to plan your shopping with confidence. You'll soon discover that not only does Food Optimising work, it's fabulously simple too!**

These menus are designed to help you understand the variety of meals that are possible when you start Food Optimising. You're sure to have plenty of nourishing food that will keep you full and healthy – and help you to lose weight. In these menus we have included some of the recipes that are low in Syns in this book. Should you want to incorporate other recipes from the book, simply include their Syn values (should there be any) in your daily allowance.

**Here's how to use Food Optimising menus most effectively:**
**1** Decide whether you wish to have a **Green** or **Original day** and stick to that choice all day. You can make every day a **Green** day or include some **Original days** too. Within the Green menus we have included meat-free choices suitable for
vegetarians.
**2** Pick one breakfast, one lunch and one dinner from your chosen set.
**3** Choose around 10 to 15 Syns-worth of food from the Syns list on page 221. Some Food Optimisers find they lose weight best on 5 Syns, others on 20 Syns. On some days, you might find you perhaps need to use 30, if you are going out or celebrating. In general, we find 10 Syns a day is a good rule of thumb for effective weight loss.
**4** Each day, choose twice from the following milk and cheese lists to boost your calcium intake, which is vital for a healthy diet.

**Milk**
- 350ml/12fl oz skimmed milk
- 250ml/8fl oz semi-skimmed milk
- 175ml/6fl oz whole milk
- 250ml/8fl oz calcium-enriched soya milk (sweetened or unsweetened)

**Cheese**
- 30g/1oz Cheddar
- 30g/1oz Edam
- 30g/1oz Gouda
- 40g/1½oz Mozzarella

- 3 triangles Original Dairylea
- 2 mini Babybel cheeses

Drink black tea, coffee (sweetened with artificial sweetener) and low-calorie drinks freely, and use fat-free French or vinaigrette-style salad dressings freely.

On the menus that are given on the following pages – divided into **Green days** and **Original days** – check out the foods that are marked in **bold**. These can be eaten freely without any weighing or measuring. Fill up on these foods when you feel peckish. You can also turn to our Free Food list on page 220 and select other Free Foods to enjoy whenever you want, in whatever quantity you want.

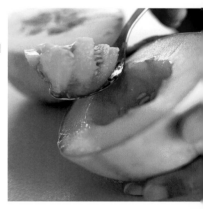

**Maximise your healthy eating by:**
- Eating at least five portions of fresh fruit and vegetables every day. Frozen and canned vegetables can also be used.
- Trimming any visible fat off meat and removing any skin from poultry.
- Varying your choices as much as possible to ensure the widest range of nutrients in your diet.
- Eating at least two portions of fish a week, of which one is an oily fish.
- Trying to avoid eating more than ten eggs per week as these are particularly high in cholesterol. People with high blood cholesterol are advised not to eat more than four eggs per week, although each individual should check with their doctor.
- Aiming to keep your salt intake to no more than 6g a day (about 1 level teaspoon). As well as limiting the amount of table salt you add to food, watch out for salt added to manufactured foods and sauces. Try flavouring foods with herbs and spices instead.
- Remembering the latest recommendations regarding intake of fluids, which is to aim for six to eight cups, mugs or glasses of any type of fluid per day (excluding alcohol).

- **Note for Slimming World members:** Healthy Extra B choices are built into the menus.

When you have experienced the pleasure of Food Optimising on your plate you will want to make your own menus. You can do this with the complete Food Optimising system, available at Slimming World groups throughout the UK.

GREEN MENUS

# Breakfasts

**1**
Fresh **melon** wedges
followed by
30g/1oz Shredded Wheat Honey Nut
served with milk from the allowance
topped with heaps of fresh
**strawberries**.

**2**
Two slices wholemeal bread,
toasted and topped with oodles of
**spaghetti hoops/baked beans**
in tomato sauce,
plus an **apple** and **banana**.

**3**
90g/3oz grilled lean bacon
(approximately 3 rashers),
poached **egg**, grilled **tomatoes**
and **mushrooms**,
plus a **peach**.

**4**
Fresh **grapefruit** sweetened with
artificial sweetener if desired,
followed by
45g/1½oz Nestlé Fibre 1
served with milk from the allowance
and a pot of **Marks & Spencer
Count on Us yogurt (any variety)**.

**5**
30g/1oz Alpen or bran flakes
topped with a pile of **blueberries**
and served with milk from the
allowance followed by
**Potato and spring onion pancakes**
(see page 46) served with poached
**eggs** and grilled **tomatoes**.

**6**
Kedgeree:
sliced **onion** fried with a little Fry
Light with a pinch of curry powder,
mixed with piles of boiled **rice**,
150g/5oz flaked poached haddock and
quartered hard boiled **egg**,
plus an **apple**.

**7**
**Club-style bean burger breakfast**
(see page 55)
followed by
an **apple, pear** and **satsumas**.

**8**
Two slices of wholemeal toast topped
with **Akuri Indian-style scrambled
eggs** (see page 52)
followed by
a **banana** and **Müllerlight yogurt**.

**9**
Yogurt crunch made with
**very low fat natural yogurt**,
30g/1oz Jordans Luxury Muesli and
sliced **kiwi**: layer the kiwi, muesli and
yogurt right to the top of a tall glass
finishing with a sprinkling of muesli
and a slice of **kiwi**,
followed by
a **banana**.

**10**
A large fluffy **omelette** filled with
grilled **mushrooms, tomatoes** and
30g/1oz grated Cheddar cheese and
served with plenty of **baked beans**,
plus a **banana**.

# Lunches

**1**
**Puy lentil salad** (see page 94)
followed by
300g/10oz blackberries,
stewed with sweetener topped with
plenty of **very low fat natural yogurt.**

**2**
**Large jacket potato** filled with
30g/1oz grated Cheddar cheese and
plenty of **baked beans** in tomato
sauce served with a huge fresh **salad.**
Plus an **apple** and **banana**.

**3**
Courgette, red pepper and mint
frittata (see page 62)
followed by 350g/12oz pears, canned
in juice, topped with a generous
serving of **very low fat natural
fromage frais**.

**4**
**Jacket potato** filled with 110g/4oz
tuna canned in brine, served with
**sweetcorn** and a generous selection
of **radicchio, endive, radishes**
and cherry **tomatoes** followed by
sliced **banana** topped with
**Müllerlight toffee yogurt** and a
sprinkling of **cinnamon**.

**5**
**Harlequin Rice Salad** (see page 92)
followed by
an abundance of **strawberries** and
**raspberries** layered with **Müllerlight
vanilla yogurt** and sprinkled with
20g/³⁄₄oz chopped mixed nuts.

**6**
Herby tabouleh salad (see page 65)
followed by
240g/8oz apple, baked and filled with
1 level tablespoon of mincemeat and
topped with plenty of **very low fat
natural fromage frais.**

**7**
60g/2oz wholemeal crusty roll filled
with sliced **eggs** and **tomato**
followed by
a big bowl of fresh
**strawberries** topped with
**very low fat natural yogurt.**

**8**
90g/3oz smoked salmon served with a
delicious Mixed grilled pepper and
basil salad (see page 84) and new
**potatoes** cooked with fresh **mint** and
tons of **salad**.

**9**
110g/4oz skinless and boneless
chicken breast, grilled and served with
a plateful of **Roasted 'al fresco'
vegetable couscous** (see page 66)
plus a **pear** and **banana**.

**10**
Pasta and prawn salad made with
**pasta** shapes, 175g/6oz prawns,
cherry **tomatoes**, chopped **peppers,
cucumber, sweetcorn** and freshly
chopped **basil** mixed with **Quark**
flavoured with freshly chopped **garlic**.
Followed by an **orange** and fresh
**cherries** and/or **grapes**.

# Dinners

**1**

Vegetable biryani (see page 174) served with **very low fat natural yogurt** and **cucumber salad** plus a large bowl of chopped **apple, pear** and **grapes** topped with plenty of **Danone Shape Truly Fruity yogurt**.

**2**

Large serving of **Middle Eastern vegetable casserole with couscous** (see page 188) plus an **apple** and **orange**.

**3**

Vegetable stir-fry: **broccoli** and **cauliflower** florets, chopped **carrots**, mixed **peppers**, **spring onions**, button **mushrooms, beansprouts** and **water chestnuts** stir-fried with **garlic, herbs** and **soy sauce** served on a generous bed of **noodles**, plus an **apple**.

**4**

Chilled summer gazpacho (see page 72) followed by **Farfalle and mixed bean salad** (see page 88) plus a refreshing bowl of fresh tropical fruit salad made with loads of chopped **mango, kiwi fruit** and **papaya**.

**5**

**Oriental mushroom pâté** with a huge selection of **crudités** (see page 68) followed by Minted asparagus risotto (see page 177) plus a **banana**.

**6**

Large **omelette** filled with chopped **peppers, red onions** and **sweetcorn**, served with **Crispy stuffed potato skins** (see page 130) and loads of **salad**. Plus half a canteloupe **melon** piled high with **raspberries**.

**7**

**Spaghetti bolognese** (see page 112) followed by a huge selection of fresh **berries** topped with spoonfuls of **very low fat natural fromage frais** flavoured with **vanilla**.

**8**

**Large jacket potato** filled with a can of mixed **beans** in a chilli sauce served with a generous mixed **salad** plus heaps of **strawberries** topped with a **Müllerlight vanilla yogurt**.

**9**

**Mild and creamy Quorn curry** (see page 113) served with mountains of boiled **rice**, plus an **apple** and **satsuma**.

**10**

Spinach and courgette cannelloni (see page 108) served with heaps of **baby whole sweetcorn** and **carrots** followed by masses of **very low fat natural fromage frais** mixed with sliced **banana** and **vanilla**.

# Breakfasts

**1**

Fresh **grapefruit** followed by loads of lean grilled **gammon**, poached **egg**, grilled **tomatoes** and **mushrooms** served with two slices of wholemeal toast.

**2**

30g/1oz Shredded Wheat Bitesize/Honey Nut cereal served with milk from the allowance and sliced **banana**, plus a generous serving of **Danone Simply Berries yogurt**.

**3**

Tons of fresh **apricots**, chopped and topped with **very low fat natural fromage frais** or **yogurt** followed by grilled lean **bacon**, scrambled **egg** and 150g/5oz baked beans in tomato sauce.

**4**

A large bowl of **orange** and **grapefruit** segments followed by a generous portion of **Herby smoked salmon scrambled eggs** (see page 54) served with grilled large flat **mushrooms** and two slices of wholemeal toast.

**5**

A big bowl of fresh **strawberries** and **melon** topped with a **Müllerlight Country Berries yogurt** followed by grilled **kippers** served with a 60g/2oz wholemeal roll.

**6**

Banana split: **banana** sliced lengthways, sprinkled with 40g/1½oz Nestlé Fibre 1 and topped with oodles of **very low fat natural yogurt**.

**7**

Two Weetabix served with milk from the allowance followed by a large fluffy **omelette** filled with lean **ham** and **mushrooms**.

**8**

Generous slices of **melon** followed by **Egg and tomato bakes with parsnip chips** (see page 48) served with lean grilled **bacon**.

**9**

Two slices of wholemeal toast topped with plum **tomatoes** with a dash of **Worcestershire sauce** followed by a **peach** or **nectarine**.

**10**

A generous serving of fresh fruit salad (e.g. **apple, pear, grapes** and **orange**), followed by **Egg and mushroom Florentines** (see page 51) served with crispy grilled lean **bacon** and two slices of wholemeal bread.

# Lunches

**1**

Fresh **tuna** or **swordfish** steak baked in the oven with **coriander** and **lemon juice** served with a large mixed **salad** and a 240g/8oz baked potato (raw weight) followed by a bunch of **grapes**.

**2**

**Pork and mushroom stroganoff** (see page 120) served with 200g/7oz new potatoes in their skins and plenty of **broccoli** and **leeks**. Plus a **banana** and **pear**.

**3**

Provençal pan-cooked chicken (see page 116) served with 100g/3$\frac{1}{2}$oz (boiled weight) wholemeal pasta and a big mixed **salad** followed by a **Müllerlight yogurt** and an **apple**.

**4**

**Spicy Thai-style beef salad** (see page 103) followed by 300g/10oz apple and 300g/10oz rhubarb, stewed and topped with lashings of **very low fat natural fromage frais**.

**5**

**Tuna, salmon or chicken** served with salad with a variety of **salad leaves**, cherry **tomatoes,** diced **cucumber**, **peppers** and **celery, spring onions** and chopped hard-boiled **egg** served with a 60g/2oz wholemeal roll, followed by **strawberries** and **melon**.

**6**

Roast **turkey** breast served with North African carrot and coriander salad (see page 91) and 200g/7oz new potatoes in their skins, followed by a **pear**.

**7**

225g/8oz jacket potato (raw weight) filled with **very low fat natural cottage cheese** and chopped **spring onions** served with lots of **salad**, plus chopped **apples** and **orange** segments topped with **very low fat natural fromage frais**.

**8**

Honey and mustard roast salmon with roasted ratatouille (see page 164) served with plenty of **broccoli, carrots, baby whole sweetcorn** and **mangetout**, followed by 400g/14oz fruit cocktail canned in juice.

**9**

Peppered roast beef with roasted root vegetables (see page 170) followed by 225g/8oz apple, baked and filled with 110g/4oz stewed blackberries.

**10**

Prawn, mango and herb salad (see page 96) served with 225g/8oz jacket potato (raw weight) or two slices of wholemeal bread followed by a **banana** and **pear**.

# Dinners

### 1
Lean fillet **steak** tossed in crushed black **peppercorns**, grilled and served with **baby whole sweetcorn, sugar snap peas** and **asparagus**. Plus a large fresh fruit salad, e.g. chopped **apple, banana** and **peach**.

### 2
**Calypso lamb steaks with Cajun tomato and red pepper sauce** (see page 189) served with **green beans** and **cabbage**, followed by heaps of **raspberries** and **strawberries** topped with **very low fat natural fromage frais.**

### 3
**Seared squid with tomato salad** (see page 181) followed by generous slices of fresh **melon**.

### 4
**Citrus and garlic roasted poussins** (see page 167) served with loads of **cauliflower** and **courgettes**, plus a **pear**.

### 5
**Prawns** sprinkled with **paprika** served on a large bed of crisp **lettuce** and **cucumber** followed by a **chicken** breast, grilled or baked, served with loads of **red cabbage, thin green beans** and **butternut squash**.

### 6
**Roasted spiced pesto chicken** (see page 166) served with a large crisp green **salad,** followed by a bowl over-flowing with **raspberries, black-berries** and **blueberries** topped with **very low fat natural fromage frais**.

### 7
Long Island Seafood Skewers with a basil and tomato dip (see page 138) followed by lean **gammon** steak, grilled, topped with fresh **pineapple** chunks served with a plateful of **salad** leaves, cherry **tomatoes, cucumber, spring onions** and grated **carrot**.

### 8
**Stuffed cabbage leaves** (see page 76) followed by grilled **cod** served with **sugar snap peas, baby whole sweetcorn** and **carrots**, plus a **peach**.

### 9
**Honeydew melon**, followed by **Oriental beef and mixed pepper stir-fry** (see page 124), followed by a bowlful of fresh **mango** and sliced seedless **grapes** topped with **very low fat natural yogurt**.

### 10
**Thai aromatic chicken stir-fry** (see page 186) served with heaps of **spinach** and **pak-choi** or a large crisp green **salad** plus a bowl of chopped **kiwi** and fresh **pineapple**.

# The Food Optimising storecupboard

**When you are Food Optimising, you need ingredients at your fingertips that will enable you to produce a variety of quick, delicious meals, and help you lose weight. A good selection of spices and flavourings, for example, is essential to create a rich palette of flavours. Use the following list as a guide to useful standbys, and shop for fresh vegetables, herbs, fish and meat as you plan your meals.**

■ **Canned products:** tuna in brine or water; crabmeat in brine or water; sweetcorn niblets; borlotti, cannellini, red kidney and butter beans; chopped tomatoes (including the variety flavoured with garlic and herbs); black olives; water chestnuts; pineapple rings and peaches in natural juice; low fat coconut milk.

■ **Cooking mediums:** spray cans of Fry Light (sunflower or olive oil based); olive oil and sesame oil (sometimes needed in tiny amounts to flavour a recipe).

■ **Spices and flavourings:** sea salt, black and mixed peppercorns; coriander, cumin, caraway and fennel seeds; allspice and juniper berries; nutmeg, star anise, cloves, cardamom, ground cinnamon and cinnamon sticks; ground cumin, coriander, paprika, ginger, mixed spice, chilli powder; tandoori spice mix; curry powder; Cajun spice seasoning, dried chilli flakes; dried herbs, such as oregano; vanilla pods; saffron strands.

■ **Jars and bottles:** Tabasco; Worcestershire sauce; sweet chilli sauce; passata; hoisin sauce; light and dark soy sauces; reduced-sugar apricot jam; Thai fish sauce; reduced-calorie mayonnaise; Dijon and wholegrain mustards; honey; capers and caperberries; gherkins; grated or creamed horseradish; mint jelly; chicken and beef Bovril; vegetable stock powder; balsamic, red and white wine vinegars; tarragon and cider vinegars.

■ **Staples:** plain and wholemeal flours; long-grain, arborio, brown and wild rice; wholemeal and regular pasta, such as penne, spaghetti, linguini, pappardelle and fusilli; noodles; couscous and bulghar wheat; red lentils.

■ **Additional items:** cornflour and arrowroot (to thicken sauces); artificial granulated sweetener; instant coffee granules; good-quality chocolate; gelatine or vegi-gel, and sugar-free jelly crystals; meringue nests.

■ **Alcohol for cooking:** red wine, dark rum, amaretto liqueur and marsala.

■ **Fridge items:** very low fat natural fromage frais, yogurt and crème fraîche; Quark soft cheese; reduced fat hard cheese; Parmesan; eggs; skimmed or semi-skimmed milk; Quorn mince and pieces.

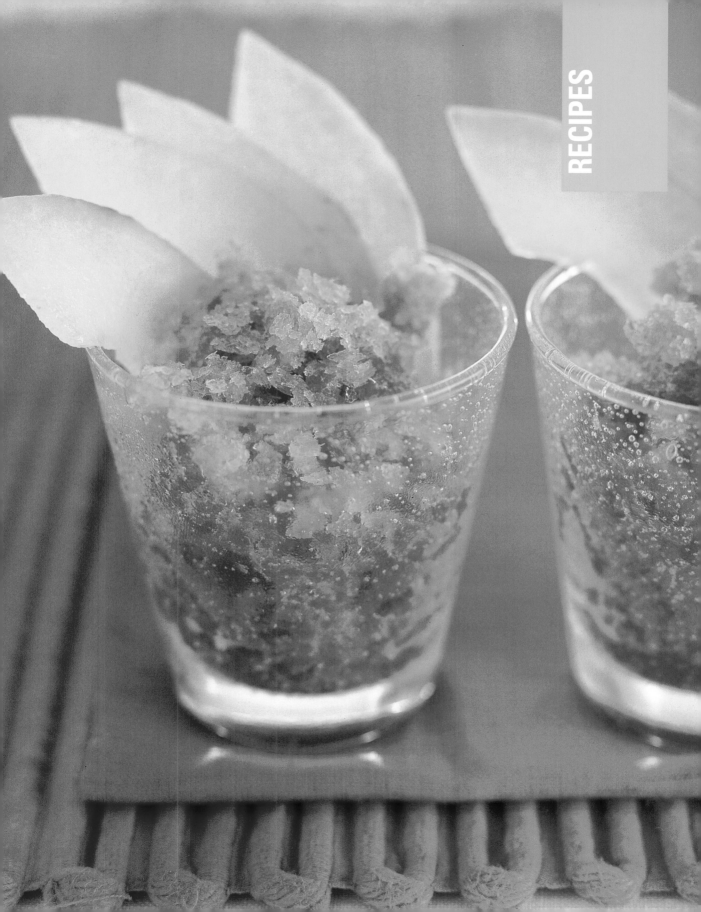

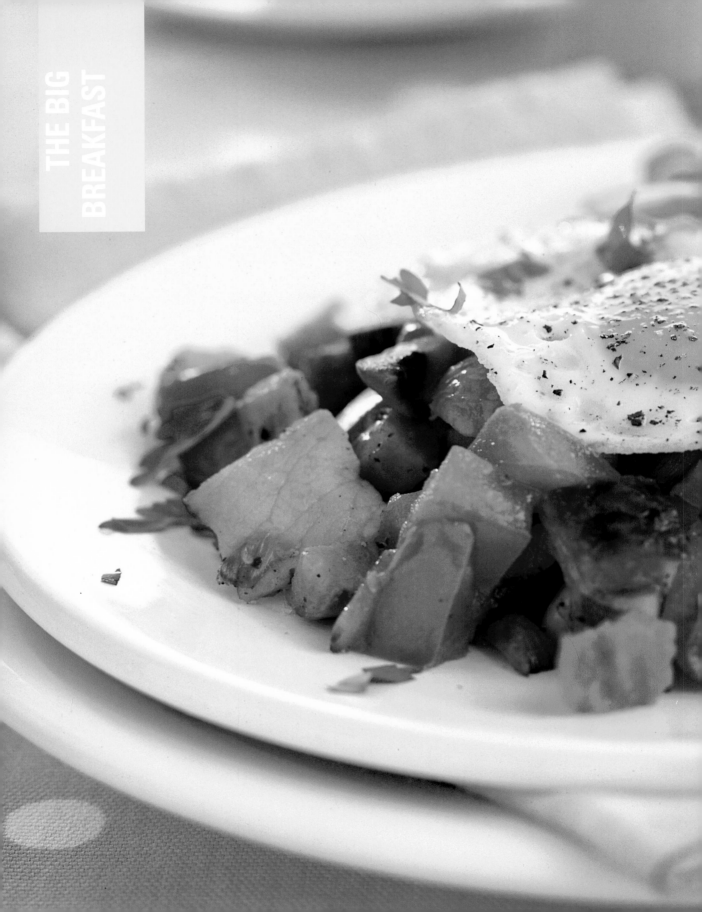

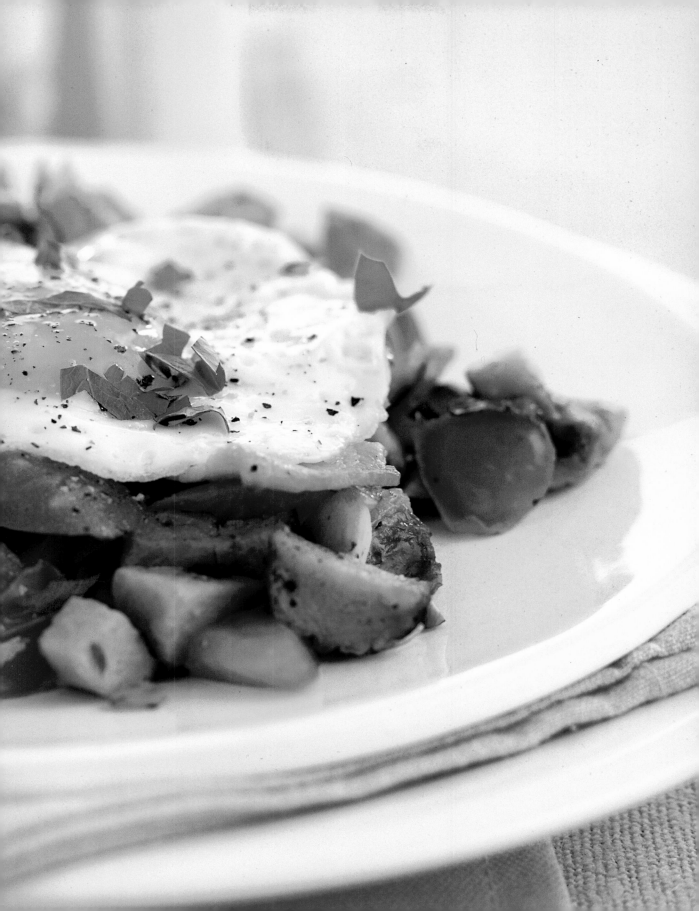

**serves** 4
**preparation time**
15 minutes
**cooking time**
12–16 minutes
**vegetarian**
**syns per serving**
original **4¹/₂**
green **4¹/₂**

GREEN/ORIGINAL

# Fruity French toast

Quick and easy to prepare, these special egg-dipped toasts are a wonderful way to start the day.

200ml/7fl oz skimmed milk
2 eggs
3–4 tbsp artificial sweetener
¹/₄ tsp ground cinnamon
a few drops of vanilla essence
4 slices white bread, thinly sliced

Fry Light for spraying
400g/14oz mixed sliced fruit
 (e.g. peaches, plums, strawberries,
 oranges)
200g/7oz very low fat natural yogurt

◼ Place the milk in a bowl and add the eggs, sweetener, cinnamon and the vanilla. Whisk until frothy and then pour into a large, shallow dish.

◼ Dip the bread slices into the milk mixture and let them soak, turning to coat both sides.

◼ Spray a large, non-stick frying pan with Fry Light and place over a medium heat. Fry the slices in batches for 2–3 minutes per side until lightly golden.

◼ To serve, cut each slice in half diagonally and place on four serving plates. Divide the berries between the plates and top with the yogurt. Serve immediately.

**BONUS POINT**
To make a savoury version of these toasts omit the sweetener, vanilla and cinnamon and add chopped herbs to the egg. Serve with tomatoes and mushrooms.

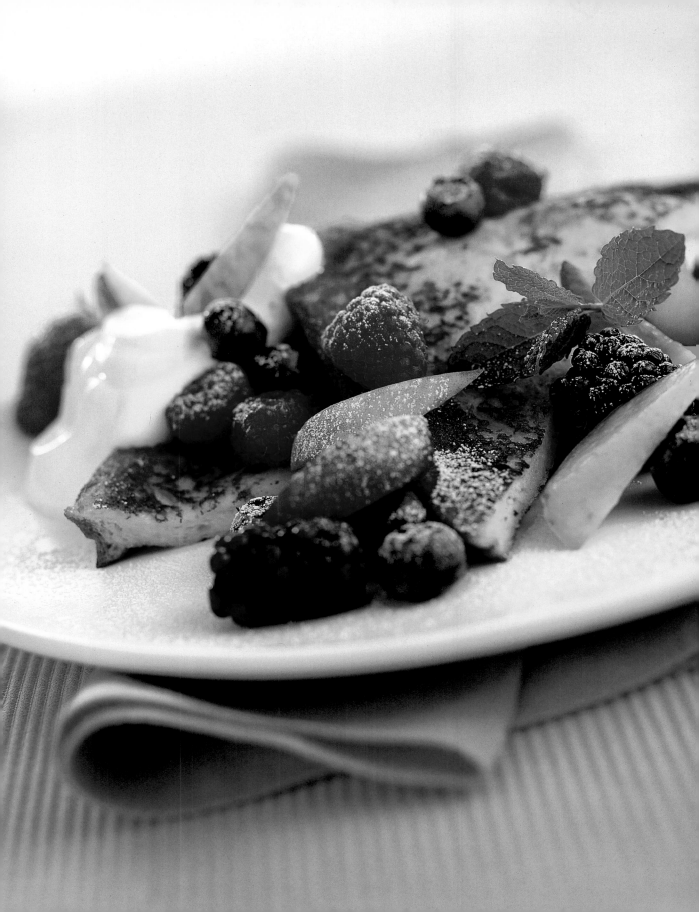

**serves** 4
**preparation time**
15 minutes
**cooking time**
12–15 minutes
**vegetarian**
**syns per serving**
original **7**
green **free**

GREEN

# Root vegetable rostis

Poached eggs can replace the soft-boiled eggs in this quick, easy and filling breakfast treat.

for the rostis:
300g/10oz potatoes, peeled
200g/7oz sweet potatoes, peeled
300g/10oz parsnips, peeled
4 spring onions, finely sliced
3 tbsp finely snipped chives

1 medium egg
salt and freshly ground black pepper
Fry Light for spraying
to serve:
4 soft-boiled eggs
4 grilled tomatoes (optional)

■ Coarsely grate the potatoes, sweet potatoes and parsnips and place in a fine metal sieve and squeeze out as much liquid as possible. Transfer to a large mixing bowl.

■ Stir in the spring onions and chives. Lightly beat the egg and stir into the mixture. Season well and mix thoroughly.

■ Preheat the oven to 200°C/Gas 6. Line a baking sheet with non-stick baking parchment and spray with Fry Light. Divide the rosti mixture into eight portions and spoon onto the prepared baking sheet, flattening each portion slightly with the back of the spoon. Bake for 12–15 minutes or until the rostis are lightly browned and cooked through.

■ To serve, place two rostis on each warmed serving plate and top with a soft-boiled egg. Accompany with grilled tomatoes if desired.

**BONUS POINT**
These rostis can be frozen for up to three months. Layer the cooked rostis between sheets of baking parchment and transfer to a freezerproof container.

# Breakfast corn slice

As eggs are Free on both the Green and Original choice, this delicious dish is low on Syns.

**serves** 4
**preparation time**
20 minutes
**cooking time**
35–40 minutes
**vegetarian**
**syns per serving**
original **1½**
green **free**

Fry Light for spraying
100g/3½oz raw sweetcorn kernels
4 large eggs
4 spring onions, finely chopped
100g/3½oz very low fat natural
 fromage frais

2 tomatoes, deseeded and finely
 chopped
2 tbsp chopped flat-leaf parsley
salt and freshly ground black pepper

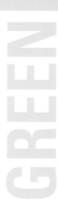

GREEN

■ Preheat the oven to 180°C/Gas 4. Lightly spray a 20cm (8in) non-stick cake tin with Fry Light and line with non-stick baking parchment.

■ Place the sweetcorn in a bowl and add the eggs. Beat lightly with a fork and stir in the spring onions, fromage frais, tomatoes and chopped parsley. Season well and pour into the tin.

■ Place the tin in the preheated oven and bake for 35–40 minutes or until the mixture is firm to the touch and set. Take out of the oven and cool for 4–5 minutes. Then carefully remove from the tin, discard the baking paper and serve, cut into wedges.

**BONUS POINT**
This dish is great eaten cold too and you can ring the changes by substituting chopped green beans for the sweetcorn.

**serves** 4
**preparation time**
15 minutes
+ chilling
**cooking time**
20–30 minutes
**vegetarian**
**syns per serving**
original **8**
green **free**

GREEN

# Potato and spring onion pancakes

This dish is Free Food on the Green choice and makes a very nourishing and tasty breakfast.

900g/2lb potatoes
4 spring onions
2 tbsp chopped parsley
salt and freshly ground black pepper
Fry Light for spraying

to serve:
4 fried (using Fry Light), poached or
   scrambled eggs
4 grilled tomatoes

▪ Scrub, peel and chop the potatoes into small pieces. Fill a large saucepan with lightly salted water and add the potatoes. Bring to the boil and cook for 12–15 minutes or until tender. Drain and return to the pan.

▪ Slice the spring onions finely and add to the potatoes. Mash the mixture until fairly smooth and then stir in the chopped parsley. Season well, cover and chill for 3–4 hours.

▪ When ready to cook, divide the potato mixture into 12 portions and form each one into a small 'pancake'.

▪ Spray a large, non-stick frying pan with Fry Light and place over a medium heat. Cook the potato pancakes in batches of two or three for 3–4 minutes on each side, or until lightly golden. Transfer to a plate lined with greaseproof paper and keep warm while you cook the remaining pancakes.

▪ Place three pancakes on each warmed serving plate and serve with the eggs of your choice and grilled tomatoes.

**BONUS POINT**
For a more zesty taste, use chives instead of the parsley.

# Crunchy fruit and yogurt breakfast bowl

This makes a healthy and easy start to the day. For extra crunch, sprinkle a roughly crumbled gingernut biscuit over the top (an extra 2$\frac{1}{2}$ Syns).

**serves** 4
**preparation time**
15 minutes
**vegetarian**
**syns per serving**
original **free**
green **free**

200g/7oz green seedless grapes
100g/3½ oz red seedless grapes
½ a small ripe pineapple
1 red apple, cored and roughly
  chopped

1 pear, cored and roughly chopped
1 tbsp lemon juice
2 x 200g/7oz pots Müllerlight vanilla-
  flavoured yogurt

■ Cut the grapes in half and place in a large mixing bowl.

■ Peel, core and chop the pineapple into bite-sized chunks and add to the grapes with the apple and pear. Stir in the lemon juice and toss to mix well.

■ Spoon the mixed fruit into four bowls. Stir the yogurt and spoon over the top of the fruit salad. Serve immediately.

FREE FOOD

**BONUS POINT**
Use any fruit for this breakfast dish and you can also vary the taste by changing the flavour of the yogurt.

**FREE FOOD**

**serves** 4
**preparation time**
20 minutes
**cooking time**
about 40 minutes
**vegetarian**
**syns per serving**
*Egg and tomato*
*bakes*
original **free**
green **free**
*Parsnip chips*
original **5½**
green **free**
*Celeriac chips*
original **free**
green **free**

# Egg and tomato bakes with parsnip chips

Use firm, ripe tomatoes in this attractive breakfast dish, which would also make a great lunch if served with some steamed greens.

for the chips:
**600g/1lb 6oz parsnips or celeriac**
**Fry Light for spraying**
**salt and freshly ground black pepper**

for the baked tomatoes:
**8 large tomatoes**
**salt**

**a small bunch of basil leaves and**
    **flat-leaf parsley**
**freshly ground black pepper**
**8 eggs**

to garnish:
**chopped flat-leaf parsley**
**salad leaves**

■ Preheat the oven to 200°C/Gas 6. Peel the parsnips or celeriac and cut into 1cm/½in thick 'fingers'. Place on a non-stick baking sheet, spray with Fry Light and season well. Bake in the oven for 15–20 minutes or until lightly browned. Remove and keep warm.

■ Turn the oven down to 180°C/Gas 4. Slice the tops off the tomatoes and scoop out the seeds using a small spoon. Discard the tomato 'lids' and lightly season the tomato insides with some salt. Place onto kitchen paper, cut side down, for 15–20 minutes.

■ Meanwhile, finely chop the basil and parsley. Line a baking sheet with non-stick baking parchment and place the tomatoes on the sheet, cut side up. Spoon in the chopped herbs and season with freshly ground black pepper.

■ Break an egg into each tomato and bake in the oven for 15–20 minutes or until the eggs are cooked to your liking. Serve immediately, garnished with chopped parsley and accompanied by the parsnip or celeriac chips.

**BONUS POINT**
The chips can be frozen after being cooked. To use, heat from frozen in a hot oven for 15–20 minutes.

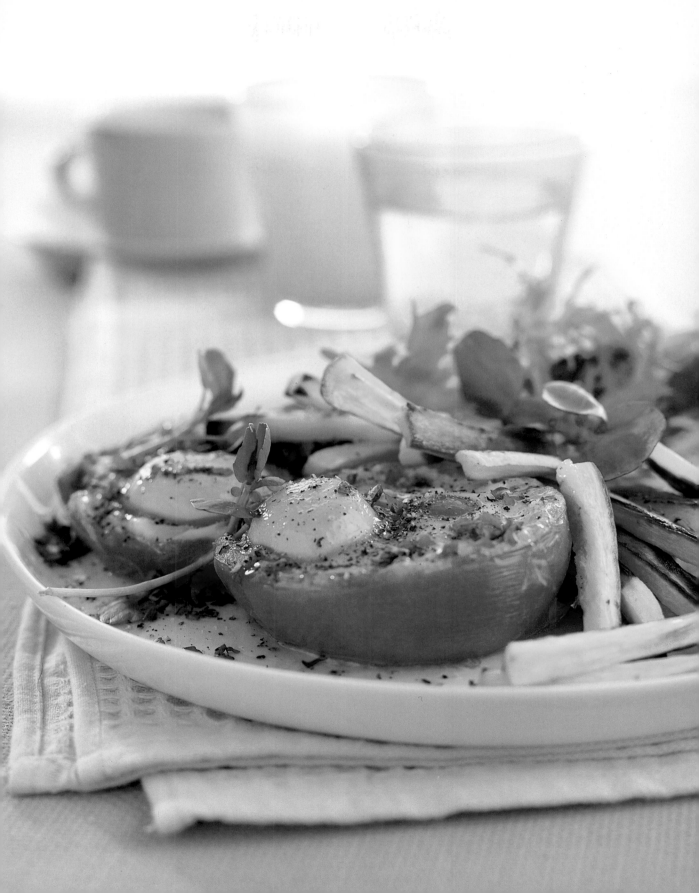

**serves** 4
**preparation time**
10 minutes
**cooking time**
6–8 minutes
**vegetarian**
**syns per serving**
original **free**
green **free**

# Asparagus dippers with soft-boiled eggs

Free Food on both choices, this simple but delicious combination of egg and asparagus makes a nutritious and tasty breakfast.

**32 thick asparagus tips**
**8 large eggs**
**salt and freshly ground black pepper**

**to serve:**
**grilled vine tomatoes**

■ Bring a large pan of lightly salted water to the boil and add the asparagus tips. Boil for 2–3 minutes and then drain. Plunge into a bowl of ice-cold water and then drain again. Set aside.

■ Fill a medium-sized saucepan with water and bring to the boil. Carefully slide in the eggs with a large spoon. Reduce the heat and simmer gently for 3–5 minutes or until cooked to your liking.

■ To serve, place two eggcups on each serving plate and fill each one with a soft-boiled egg. Carefully cut off the top of each egg with a sharp knife. Place eight asparagus spears on each plate, season and use as dippers for the eggs.

**BONUS POINT**
When in season, try using thick white asparagus as an alternative to the green spears.

# Egg and mushroom florentines

For a more exotic flavour in this hearty, Free breakfast, substitute mixed wild mushrooms for the button mushrooms.

serves 4
preparation time
15 minutes
cooking time
15–20 minutes
vegetarian
syns per serving
original free
green free

1–2 tsp white wine vinegar
4 large eggs
Fry Light for spraying
400g/14oz button mushrooms, roughly chopped
½ onion, peeled and finely chopped

60ml/2fl oz vegetable stock
100g/3½oz spinach leaves, finely chopped
salt and freshly ground black pepper

■ Bring a large pan of lightly salted water to the boil. Stir in the vinegar, reduce the heat to a very gentle simmer and carefully break the eggs into the water. Cover the pan and let the eggs poach on a very low heat for about 4 minutes. Remove from the heat and carefully transfer the eggs to a large bowl of cold water.

■ Spray a large, non-stick frying pan with Fry Light and place over a high heat. Add the mushrooms and then the onions and stir-fry for 4–5 minutes. Add the stock and the spinach leaves and cook for 3–4 minutes. Season well.

■ Divide the mushroom mixture between four warmed plates and then carefully place a poached egg on top of each serving. Season and serve immediately.

FREE FOOD

**BONUS POINT**
If you are having an Original day, top the dish with some crispy grilled lean bacon.

**serves** 4
**preparation time**
15 minutes
**cooking time**
about 8 minutes
**vegetarian**
**syns per serving**
original **free**
green **free**

# Akuri Indian-style scrambled eggs

A scrambled egg with an interesting and flavoursome twist, this piquant breakfast dish will put a spark to any cold winter morning.

2 plum tomatoes
½ small red onion
4–5 tbsp chopped coriander
  leaves
9 eggs
a pinch of turmeric
a pinch of ground cumin

a pinch of ground coriander
salt and freshly ground black pepper
Fry Light for spraying

to serve:
100g/3½oz watercress
chopped coriander leaves

■  Deseed and finely chop the tomatoes. Peel and very finely chop the red onion and mix together with the tomatoes and coriander.

■  Break the eggs into a large bowl and lightly beat, adding the turmeric, cumin and coriander. Add the tomato mixture and stir well. Season to taste.

■  Spray a non-stick frying pan with Fry Light and place over a medium heat. Add the egg mixture, stir and reduce the heat. Let cook undisturbed for 2–3 minutes and then, using a wooden spoon, stir and cook gently for 3–4 minutes until the eggs start to scramble and set (or until cooked to your liking). Remove from the heat.

■  To serve, divide the watercress between four warmed plates and top each plate with the scrambled eggs and serve immediately, sprinkled with chopped coriander leaves.

**BONUS POINT**
This dish makes a great sandwich filler.

52

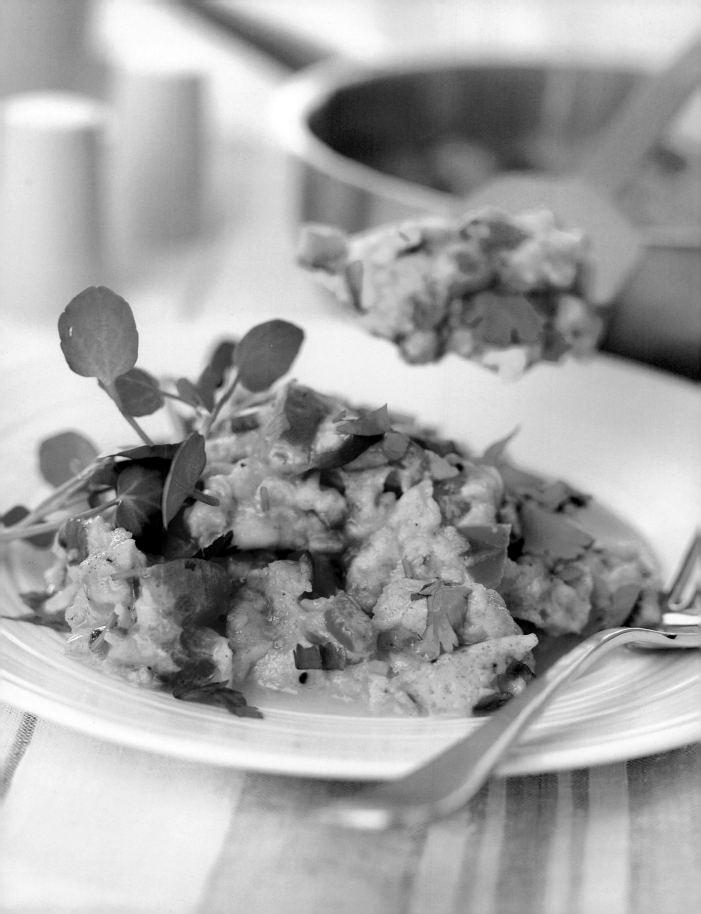

ORIGINAL

**serves** 4
**preparation time**
10 minutes
**cooking time**
6–7 minutes
**syns per serving**
original **free**
green **2**

# Herby smoked salmon scrambled eggs

The ultimate luxurious Sunday breakfast, this creamy dish of dill-flavoured scrambled eggs perfectly complements the smoked salmon.

**9 eggs**
**salt and freshly ground black pepper**
**3 tbsp finely snipped chives**
**2 tbsp finely chopped dill**
**4 x 30g/1oz slices of smoked salmon**
**Fry Light for spraying**

**to serve:**
**lemon wedges**
**sprigs of dill**
**grilled flat mushrooms**

Break the eggs into a large bowl. Lightly beat using a fork and then season well and stir in the snipped chives and dill.

Cut each slice of smoked salmon into long, thin strips and set aside.

Spray a non-stick frying pan with Fry Light and place over a medium heat. Add the egg mixture, reduce the heat and let cook for 2–3 minutes, undisturbed.

Using a wooden fork or spoon, gently stir for 2–3 minutes or until softly scrambled and just beginning to set (or until cooked to your liking). Remove the pan from the heat, stir and divide the mixture between four warmed serving plates. Top each serving with the strips of smoked salmon and serve immediately, garnished with lemon wedges and sprigs of dill and accompanied by grilled flat mushrooms.

**BONUS POINT**
For a change, smoked trout or halibut can be substituted for the salmon.

# Club-style bean burger breakfast

These delicious vegetarian burgers are excellent filling fare for breakfast … or lunch … or in the evening.

**serves** 4
**preparation time** 15 minutes + chilling
**cooking time** about 16 minutes
**vegetarian**
**syns per serving** original **11½** green **6**

**for the burgers:**
1 onion, peeled and finely chopped
1 small egg, beaten
2 tsp paprika
1 garlic clove, peeled and crushed
1 tsp ground ginger
1 tsp ground cumin
1 x 200g/7oz can chickpeas, drained and roughly mashed
1 x 200g/7oz can black-eyed beans, drained and roughly mashed

350g/12oz Quorn mince
3 tbsp finely chopped coriander leaves
salt and freshly ground black pepper
Fry Light for spraying

**to serve:**
4 x 60g/2oz wholemeal rolls
4 tomato slices
60g/2oz very low fat natural yogurt
4 small eggs, fried in Fry Light

GREEN

■ Mix the onions, egg, paprika, garlic, ground spices, chickpeas and black-eyed beans in a bowl. Add the Quorn mince and coriander, season and stir well using your fingers and divide the mixture into eight portions. Chill for 1–2 hours in the fridge.

■ When ready to cook, shape each portion into a burger and spray on both sides with Fry Light. Cook in a non-stick frying pan over a medium heat for 6–8 minutes on each side until browned and cooked through. Handle gently as the burgers are quite soft in texture.

■ To serve, split each roll in half and place a slice of tomato on the base and top with two burgers. Drizzle a little yogurt over the burgers and top each burger stack with a fried egg. Serve topped with the lid of each roll.

**BONUS POINT**
Once cooked, these burgers can successfully be frozen for up to a month.

# Pick-me-up breakfast hash

**serves** 4
**preparation time**
20 minutes
**cooking time**
about 30
minutes
**syns per serving**
original **3**
green **11**
(using Bowyers
95% fat-free
sausages)

A filling and satisfying meal, this traditional breakfast fry-up is perfect for 'the morning after'.

12 Bowyers 95% fat-free sausages
Fry Light for spraying
1 small onion, peeled and very finely
  chopped
4 rashers lean bacon (all visible fat
  removed)
200g/7oz button mushrooms,
  roughly chopped

6 plum tomatoes, deseeded and
  roughly chopped
a few drops Worcestershire sauce
salt and freshly ground black pepper
4 large eggs

to garnish:
chopped flat-leaf parsley

Chop the sausages into bite-sized pieces. Heat a large, non-stick frying pan and lightly spray with Fry Light. Add the onions and cook gently for 3–4 minutes, stirring occasionally. Add the sausages and rashers and continue to stir and fry for 3–4 minutes over a medium high heat. Add the mushrooms, tomatoes, Worcestershire sauce and seasoning and cook over a medium heat, stirring often, for 8–10 minutes. Remove the contents from the pan and keep warm.

In a separate large, non-stick frying pan, lightly sprayed with Fry Light, fry the eggs until cooked to your liking.

To serve, divide the hash between four warmed plates and top each portion with a fried egg. Sprinkle over chopped parsley to garnish and serve immediately.

**BONUS POINT**
For some added
spice, add a dash
of Tabasco or hot
sauce to the pan.

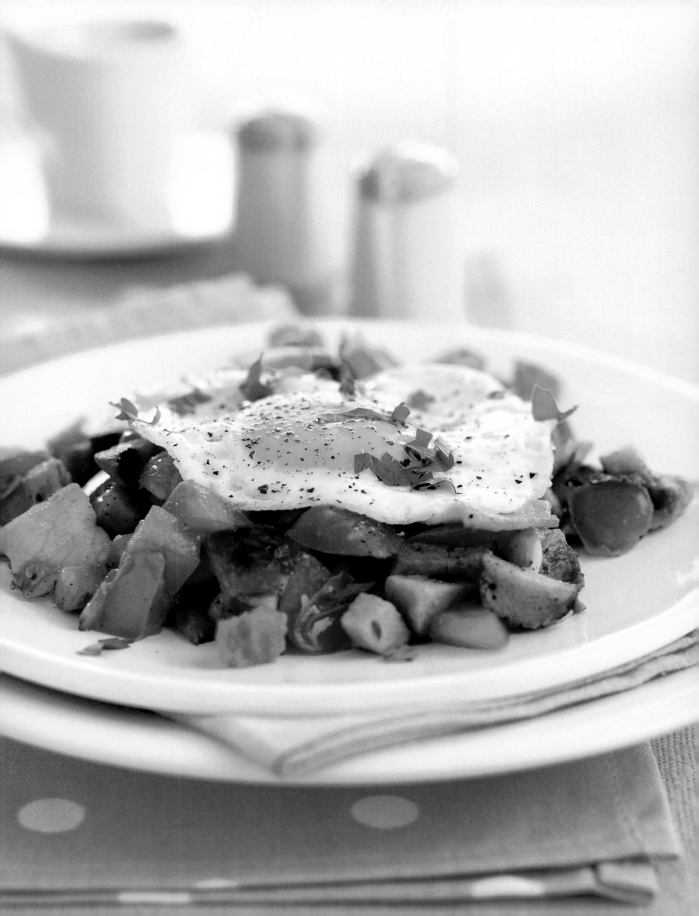

**serves** 4
**preparation time**
5 minutes
**cooking time**
about 20 minutes
**syns per serving**
original **6¹/₂**
green **3¹/₂**

# Smoked salmon kedgeree

This dish from the Raj is given an unusual twist by using smoked salmon instead of smoked haddock.

150g/5oz easy cook Basmati rice
1 red onion, peeled and finely
   chopped
60ml/2fl oz stock made from Bovril
1 tbsp mild curry powder
a pinch of turmeric
1 tsp ground ginger
4 hard-boiled eggs

4 tbsp chopped parsley
200g/7oz smoked salmon, roughly
   chopped
salt and freshly ground black pepper

to serve:
wedges of lemon

■ Cook the rice according to the packet instructions, drain and set aside.

■ Place the onion and stock in a non-stick frying pan and bring to the boil. Reduce the heat and add the curry powder, turmeric and ground ginger. Stir to mix well and then add the drained, cooked rice and stir to mix well once again.

■ Roughly chop the hard-boiled eggs and add to the rice mixture with the chopped parsley and smoked salmon. Remove from the heat, season well and serve immediately with lemon wedges.

**BONUS POINT**
For a healthier option, use brown Basmati rice instead of the more usual white.

# Minted summer fruit vanilla smoothie

Breakfast in a glass … this healthy, colourful and vibrant drink is low in Syns – and full of goodness.

**serves** 4
**preparation time**
10 minutes
**vegetarian**
**syns per serving**
original **1½**
green **1½**

**100g/3½ oz strawberries**
**100g/3½ oz raspberries**
**100g/3½ oz blueberries**
**100g/3½ oz blackberries**
**1 tbsp very finely chopped mint leaves**
**6 tbsp artificial sweetener**
**a few drops of vanilla extract**

**450g/1lb very low fat natural yogurt**
**100ml/3½fl oz chilled water**

**to garnish:**
**a few berries**

Place the strawberries, raspberries, blueberries and blackberries in a food processor with the chopped mint, sweetener, vanilla, yogurt and chilled water.

Process for 1–2 minutes or until smooth and frothy.

Pour into four chilled glasses and serve immediately, garnished with a few berries.

**BONUS POINT**
If you feel like a change, use mangoes and apricots instead of the berries.

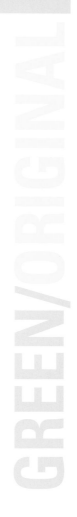
GREEN/ORIGINAL

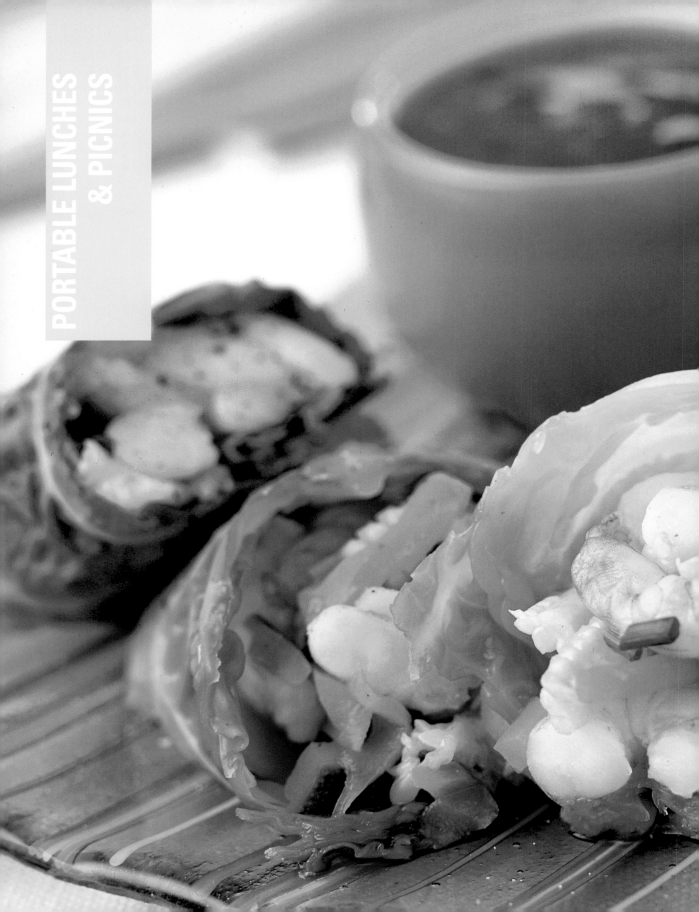

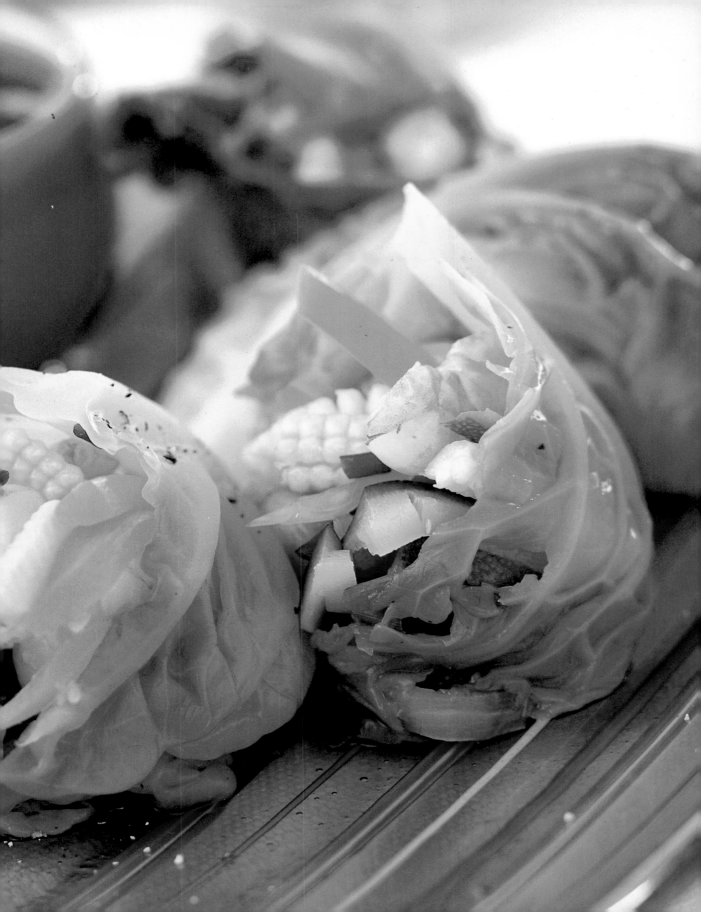

serves 4
**preparation time**
15 minutes
**cooking time**
about 30 minutes
**vegetarian**
**syns per serving**
original **1**
green **1**

# Courgette, red pepper and mint frittata

Perfect picnic fare, this frittata is delicious when eaten hot or if allowed to cool to room temperature.

Fry Light for spraying
**6–8 spring onions, finely sliced**
**2 courgettes, cut into 1cm/½ in**
  **pieces**
**1 red pepper, deseeded and cut into**
  **1cm/½ in pieces**
**6 eggs**

**3 tbsp finely chopped mint leaves**
**1 tbsp finely chopped flat-leaf parsley**
**salt and freshly ground black pepper**
**2 level tbsp grated Parmesan cheese**

to serve:
**mixed salad leaves**

■ Spray a medium-sized, non-stick frying pan with Fry Light and place over a high heat. Add the spring onions, courgettes and red pepper and stir-fry for 6–8 minutes until lightly browned and just tender.

■ Break the eggs into a bowl, lightly beat and add the chopped herbs. Season well and pour over the vegetables in the frying pan. Turn the heat to low, cover and cook gently for 12–15 minutes.

■ Heat the grill to medium. Uncover the frying pan, sprinkle with the Parmesan cheese and grill for 4–5 minutes or until the frittata is just set and the top is golden. Remove from the grill and allow to cool before cutting into wedges and serve with a mixed leaf salad.

**BONUS POINT**
This frittata can be made up to two days in advance, wrapped in cling film and chilled until ready to use.

**GREEN/ORIGNAL**

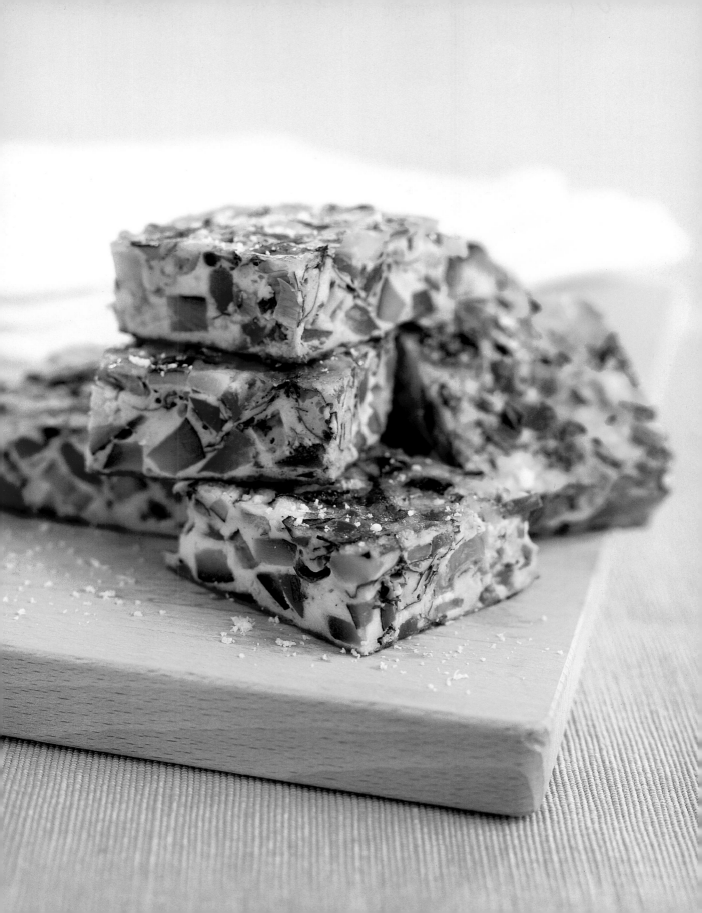

serves 4
**preparation time**
10 minutes
**cooking time**
12 minutes
**vegetarian**
**syns per serving**
original **12**
green **½**

GREEN

# West coast sunshine pasta salad

This salad contains the most refreshing of ingredients and it is incredibly easy to put together – just right for a lazy summer's day.

250g/9oz dried pasta shapes, e.g. shells, fusilli, farfalle

for the dressing:
juice of 2 oranges
2 tbsp red wine vinegar
1 tsp wholegrain mustard
salt and freshly ground black pepper

150g/5oz fresh pineapple, cut into bite-sized cubes
1 large orange, peeled, deseeded and cut into segments
150g/5oz green seedless grapes, halved
1 cucumber, roughly chopped
1 carrot, peeled and coarsely grated
4 spring onions, thinly sliced
a bunch of chives, snipped

■ Cook the pasta according to the packet instructions. Drain and place in a shallow salad bowl.

■ To make the dressing, mix together all the ingredients and pour over the drained pasta.

■ Add the fruit, vegetables and chopped chives to the pasta mixture and toss to mix well. Serve at room temperature.

**BONUS POINT**
This salad can be made up to a few hours in advance and chilled until ready to use. Bring to room temperature before serving.

# Herby tabbouleh salad

Free Food on a Green day, bulgur wheat is a healthy wholewheat grain widely used in Middle Eastern and Mediterranean cuisine.

**serves** 4
**preparation time** 10 minutes
**cooking time** 10 minutes
**vegetarian**
**syns per serving**
original **12**
green **1/2**

**150g/5oz bulgur wheat**
**3 large oranges**
**1 red onion, roughly chopped or cut into rings**
**4 vine tomatoes, roughly chopped**
**1 cucumber, roughly chopped**
**1 x 200g/7oz can red kidney beans, drained**
**1 x 200g/7oz can chickpeas, drained**
**a small bunch of coriander leaves, finely chopped**
**a small bunch of mint leaves, finely chopped**

**a small bunch of flat-leaf parsley, finely chopped**

for the dressing:
**juice of 2 oranges**
**juice of 1 lemon**
**1 tsp ground cumin**
**1 tsp ground ginger**
**1 clove garlic, peeled and crushed**
**salt and freshly ground black pepper**

to serve:
**lettuce leaves**
**extra herbs (optional)**

■ Cook the bulgur wheat according to the packet instructions and set aside. Place in a sieve and squeeze dry then transfer to a wide bowl. Peel the oranges with a sharp knife and cut into segments, over a bowl, saving any juices.

■ Add the orange segments, onion, tomatoes, cucumber, red kidney beans, chickpeas and chopped herbs to the bulgur wheat and toss to mix well.

■ To make the dressing, mix together all the ingredients along with the saved orange juice. Then season and pour over the salad, tossing to mix.

■ To serve, arrange the lettuce leaves on four serving plates and pile on the salad, garnishing with herbs, if desired.

**GREEN**

**BONUS POINT**
This salad is perfect picnic fare as it is extremely easy to transport.

**serves** 4
**preparation time**
25 minutes +
coucous cooling
time
**cooking time**
20–25 minutes
**vegetarian**
**syns per serving**
original **9**
green **free**

# GREEN

## Roasted 'al fresco' vegetable couscous

A wonderful dish for entertaining family and friends, this colourful couscous salad is Free Food on a Green day.

200g/7oz couscous
400g/14oz cherry tomatoes
2 red peppers, deseeded and cut into
   bite-sized pieces
2 courgettes, cut into bite-sized
   cubes
1 aubergine, cut into bite-sized cubes
3 red onions, peeled and quartered

Fry Light for spraying
salt and freshly ground black pepper
juice of 2 lemons
1 garlic clove, peeled and crushed
a large handful of basil leaves
5–6 tbsp roughly chopped flat-leaf
   parsley
2 tbsp caperberries

■ Place the couscous in a large bowl and just cover with boiling water. Cover tightly with cling film and leave it to stand for 15–20 minutes. Uncover and lightly fork the couscous to separate the grains. Set aside and cool.

■ Preheat the oven to 220°C/Gas 7. Mix together the vegetables. Spray two large, non-stick baking trays with Fry Light and spread the mixed vegetables on them in a single layer. Spray the vegetables with Fry Light and season well. Roast in the oven for 20–25 minutes until the vegetables are just tender and lightly browned. Remove and add to the prepared couscous, with all the cooking juices. Allow to cool.

■ Meanwhile, mix together the lemon juice and garlic and stir into the couscous mixture with the basil leaves, chopped parsley and caper-berries. Season and allow to cool before serving.

**BONUS POINT**
This salad can be made up to two days in advance. Just bring to room temperature before serving.

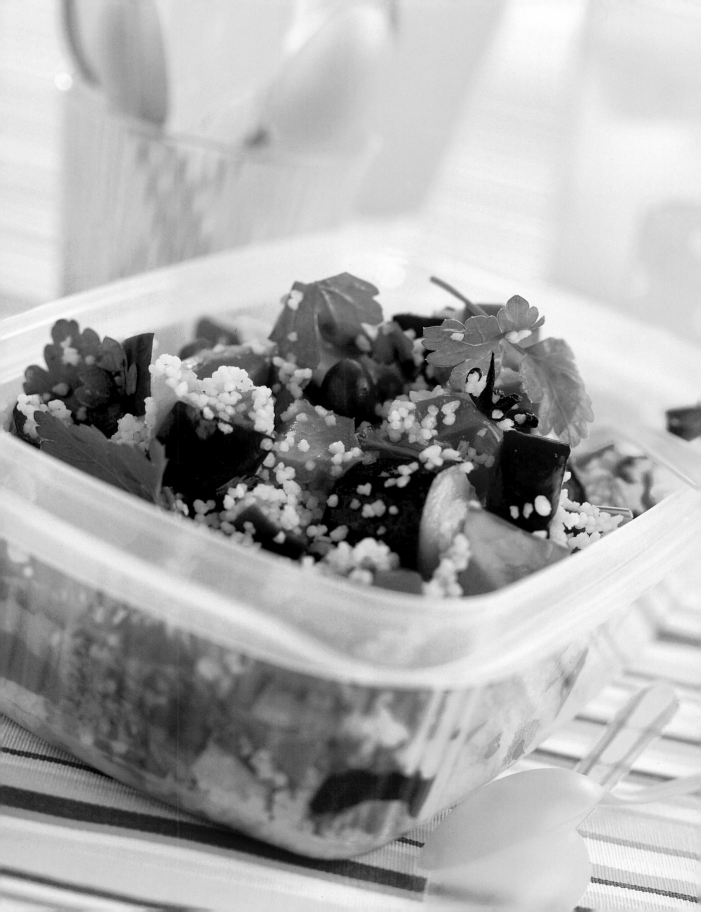

serves 4
**preparation time**
10 minutes
**cooking time**
about 15 minutes
**vegetarian**
**syns per serving**
original **free**
green **free**

# Oriental mushroom pâté with crudités

Free Food on both Green and Original days, this creamy pâté is a perfect addition to a picnic basket or even as a starter to a dinner party.

Fry Light for spraying
1 red onion, peeled and very finely chopped
1 tsp grated fresh ginger
1 tsp finely chopped lemongrass
2 garlic cloves, peeled and finely chopped
1 red chilli, deseeded and finely chopped
100g/3½ oz shiitake mushrooms, finely chopped

250g/9oz portobello mushrooms, finely chopped
100g/3½ oz Quark soft cheese
3 tbsp finely chopped coriander leaves
salt and freshly ground black pepper

to serve:
crudités, e.g. carrot, celery and cucumber batons

■ Spray a large, non-stick frying pan with Fry Light and place over a medium heat. Add the onion, ginger, lemongrass, garlic and chilli and stir-fry for 2–3 minutes.

■ Increase the heat and add the mushrooms and stir-fry for 5–6 minutes until softened. Remove from the heat and leave to cool.

■ When cool, transfer the mixture to a food processor with the Quark and coriander. Season well and blend until fairly smooth. Spoon into a bowl or individual ramekins and serve with the vegetable crudités.

**BONUS POINT**
This pâté can be made a couple of hours in advance and chilled. It can be used straight from the fridge as it doesn't have to be served at room temperature.

# Fragrant stuffed vine leaves

Perfect finger food for an outdoor event, these parcels of flavoured rice wrapped in vine leaves benefit from being made in advance.

**serves** 4
**preparation time**
20 minutes +
soaking
**cooking time**
1½ hours
**vegetarian**
**syns per serving**
original **4½**
green **free**

175g/6oz vine leaves in brine
100g/3½ oz dried Basmati rice
4 spring onions, finely sliced
2 plum tomatoes, finely chopped
1 garlic clove, peeled and crushed
2 tbsp finely chopped mint leaves

2 tbsp finely chopped flat-leaf parsley
1 tsp toasted cumin seeds
¼ tsp ground cinnamon
salt and freshly ground black pepper
2 lemons, thinly sliced

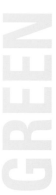

GREEN

■  Fill a large bowl with hot water and place the vine leaves in it for 30 minutes. Carefully remove and pat dry on kitchen paper.

■  Meanwhile, in a separate bowl soak the rice in boiling hot water for 5 minutes. Drain well and return to the bowl with the spring onions, tomatoes, garlic, mint, parsley, cumin seeds and cinnamon. Season well.

■  Lay the vine leaves on a clean work surface and spoon a little of the filling into the centre of each one. Fold over the sides and then roll up to encase the filling, making a 'sausage' shape.

■  Line the base of a large, non-stick saucepan with the lemon slices and place the stuffed vine leaves to fit snugly in a single layer. Cover with water and place an upturned plate over them. Cover the saucepan tightly and cook over a gentle heat for about 1½ hours, checking often that there is enough water to cover the stuffed vine leaf parcels, adding more hot water if necessary.

■  Leave the parcels to cool and then remove from the pan and chill until required.

**BONUS POINT**
If going on a picnic, fill a plastic container with shredded leaves and place the vine leaf parcels on top. Cover tightly and then they're ready to go.

**serves** 4
**preparation time**
20 minutes +
chilling
**cooking time**
12–15 minutes
**vegetarian**
**syns per serving**
original **6**
green **1/2**

# Spicy chickpea balls with yogurt relish

Perfect portable fare, these delicious morsels are so easy for all your family and friends to pick up with their fingers and pop into their mouths.

1 x 400g/14oz can chickpeas, drained
4 spring onions, finely chopped
2 garlic cloves, peeled and chopped
1 tsp finely grated ginger
2 tsp ground cumin
1 tsp ground coriander
1 tsp finely grated lime zest
1/2 tsp mild chilli powder
1 red chilli, deseeded and finely
  chopped
3 tbsp chopped coriander leaves

1/4 tsp baking powder
1/2 a small egg, lightly beaten
salt and freshly ground black pepper
Fry Light for spraying

for the relish:
1 tbsp mint jelly
200g/7oz very low fat natural yogurt
4 tbsp chopped mint leaves

■ Place the chickpeas in a sieve and rinse well. Drain and place in a food processor. Add the spring onions and garlic to the chickpeas with the ginger, ground cumin, ground coriander, lime zest, chilli powder, red chilli, fresh coriander, baking powder and the egg. Season and blend until fairly smooth. Transfer the mixture to a container, cover and chill for 3–4 hours, or overnight if time permits.

■ Preheat the oven to 200°C/Gas 6. Line a baking sheet with non-stick baking parchment and spray with Fry Light. Take small pieces of the chickpea mixture and form them into small, bite-sized balls. Place on the baking sheet and bake for 12–15 minutes or until golden and crisp.

■ Meanwhile, in a small bowl, mix together the ingredients for the relish, then season and chill until needed. Serve the chickpea balls at room temperature accompanied by the minted yogurt relish.

**BONUS POINT**
These balls can be frozen for up to a month. When you want to eat them, heat thoroughly in the oven and allow to cool before eating.

# Jewelled vegetable picnic paella

Paella makes a delicious and hearty dish. Traditionally made with Valencia rice, here it is made with brown Basmati for a healthier option.

**serves** 4
**preparation time**
15 minutes
**cooking time**
about 30 minutes
**vegetarian**
**syns per serving**
original **18¹/₂**
green **free**

350g/12oz easy-cook brown Basmati rice
a large pinch of saffron strands
200g/7oz parsnips, peeled and diced
2 carrots, peeled and diced
1 small head of broccoli, cut into small florets
Fry Light for spraying
1 large red onion, peeled and finely chopped
1 bay leaf

2 garlic cloves, peeled and crushed
200g/7oz frozen peas
100g/3¹/₂ oz baby button mushrooms
1 red chilli, deseeded and chopped
1 tsp sweet smoked paprika
salt and freshly ground black pepper

to garnish:
chopped flat-leaf parsley

**GREEN**

■ Cook the rice, along with the saffron, according to the packet instructions in a large pan of boiling water. Drain and set aside.

■ Place the parsnips, carrots and broccoli in a saucepan, cover with lightly salted water and bring to the boil. Simmer for 10–15 minutes until just tender and drain, reserving 100ml/3¹/₂fl oz of the water.

■ Spray a large, non-stick frying pan with Fry Light and add the onion, bay leaf, garlic, peas, mushrooms and red chilli. Add the reserved liquid and cook over a high heat for 10 minutes until the vegetables have softened. Add the paprika and the cooked vegetables and rice to the pan and stir to mix well. Let cool, and then pack into a picnic container together with the garnish of chopped parsley.

**BONUS POINT**
So the garnish stays fresh, pack it in a separate container and sprinkle over the paella just before serving.

**serves** 4
**preparation time**
15 minutes
+ chilling
**vegetarian**
**syns per serving**
original **1/2**
green **1/2**

# Chilled summer gazpacho

A perfect answer to a hot summer's day, this refreshing chilled soup is very straightforward to make.

900g/2lb ripe plum tomatoes
1 red pepper, deseeded and cut into chunks
2 spring onions, very finely sliced
1 cucumber, finely diced
200ml/7fl oz passata
2 garlic cloves, peeled and crushed
a few drops of Tabasco sauce
2 tbsp artificial sweetener

salt and freshly ground black pepper
1 slice Nimble wholemeal bread, crust removed
a small handful of torn basil leaves
1 tbsp white wine vinegar

to serve:
ice cubes

◼ Skin the tomatoes by making a little cross with a sharp knife in the base of each one and place them in a bowl of boiling hot water. After 1–2 minutes, remove and slip off the skins. Cut the tomatoes in half, discard the seeds and place the flesh in a food processor with the red pepper, spring onions, cucumber and passata and 200ml/7fl oz ice-cold water.

◼ Add the garlic, Tabasco, sweetener and seasoning. Roughly tear the bread and add to the mixture and then process until fairly smooth. (If you have time at this stage, you can chill the soup in the fridge for 3–4 hours.)

◼ Transfer the gazpacho to a large jug and stir in the basil and white wine vinegar. To serve, fill ice-cold bowls or wide mugs with ice and pour the gazpacho over the top.

**BONUS POINT**
For picnicing, fill a Thermos flask with ice cubes and then add the gazpacho.

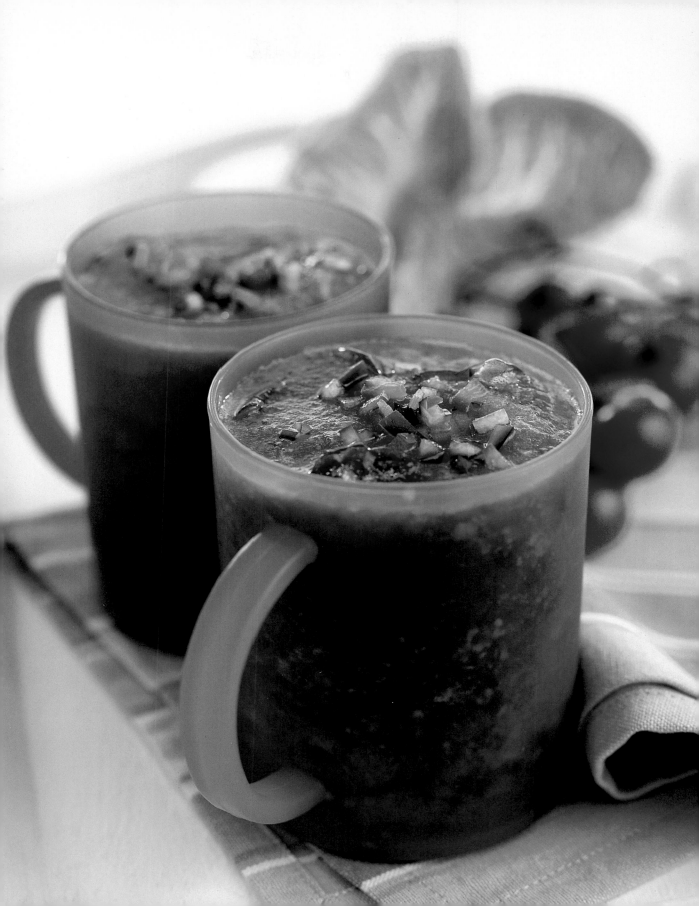

**GREEN**

serves 4
**preparation time**
20 minutes
**cooking time**
about 30 minutes
**syns per serving**
original **2**
green **1/2**

# Vichyssoise

A wonderfully versatile soup … you can serve it chilled in the summer or on a cold day heat it and serve hot.

400g/14oz leeks
200g/7oz potatoes
Fry Light for spraying
1 garlic clove, peeled and crushed
1 bay leaf
800ml/1¼pt chicken stock made
   from Bovril
100ml/3½fl oz skimmed milk

a pinch of freshly grated nutmeg
4 tbsp finely snipped chives
salt and freshly ground black pepper

to serve:
ice cubes (if serving chilled)

■ Wash and clean the leeks thoroughly, making sure to get rid of any soil or dirt. Slice them very finely and set aside.

■ Peel the potatoes and cut into small chunks.

■ Spray a large, non-stick saucepan with Fry Light and place over a medium heat. Add the leeks and potatoes and stir-fry for 3–4 minutes. Add the garlic, bay leaf and chicken stock and bring to the boil. Reduce the heat and simmer gently for 20 minutes. Discard the bay leaf.

■ Transfer the soup to a food processor and blend until smooth. Return to the saucepan and pour in the milk and 100ml/3½fl oz water and bring to the boil. Add the nutmeg and chives, then season and take off the heat. The soup can be served hot (if it is to be taken on a picnic, pour into a Thermos flask) or chilled.

■ To serve chilled, let the soup cool down, then place in the fridge for a couple of hours. To take on a picnic, fill a Thermos flask with ice cubes and pour the chilled soup over them.

**BONUS POINT**
To make the soup more fragrant, use chopped mint and coriander leaves in place of the chives.

# Dill, lemon and tuna dip

This quick and easy dip is a truly successful combination of tuna fish, dill and creamy cottage cheese, perfect for a summer picnic basket.

serves 4
**preparation time**
10 minutes +
chilling
**syns per serving**
original **free**
green **5**

**for the dip:**
2 x 185g/6½ oz cans tuna in water or
  brine
300g/10oz very low fat natural
  cottage cheese
150g/5oz very low fat natural
  fromage frais
4 spring onions, finely sliced
4 tbsp finely chopped dill

finely grated zest and juice of
  1 lemon
salt and freshly ground black pepper

**to serve:**
vegetable crudités, e.g. cauliflower
  and broccoli florets, red radishes,
  cucumbers, red and yellow peppers
hard-boiled quails' eggs

■  Drain the cans of tuna and place in a food processor.

■  Add the remaining ingredients and seasoning and blend until smooth. Transfer to a bowl and chill until ready to use.

■  Serve the dip with the vegetable crudités and quails' eggs.

ORIGINAL

**BONUS POINT**
You could always substitute canned red salmon for the tuna.

PORTABLE LUNCHES & PICNICS

# Stuffed cabbage leaves

Eaten hot or cold, these colourful and delicious parcels are best consumed by hand.

**serves** 4
**preparation time**
25 minutes
**cooking time**
8–10 minutes
**syns per serving**
original **free**
green **2**
**to serve**
soy sauce **free**
chilli sauce **½**
**per level tbsp**

ORIGINAL

**8 large Savoy cabbage leaves**
**1 courgette, cut into thin batons**
**1 carrot, peeled and cut into thin batons**
**60g/2oz baby corn, thinly sliced lengthways**
**150g/5oz cooked peeled prawns**
**4 tbsp finely chopped chives**

**½ tsp ground ginger**
**1 tsp garlic salt**
**salt and freshly ground black pepper**

**to serve:**
**soy and chilli sauces**

◼ Place the cabbage leaves in a large pan of lightly salted boiling water. Blanch for 2–3 minutes and transfer to a bowl of iced water. Drain and pat dry on kitchen paper.

◼ Mix together the courgette and carrot batons with the sliced baby corn, prawns and chives. Sprinkle over the ground ginger and garlic salt. Season and toss to mix well.

◼ Spread out the blanched cabbage leaves on a clean work surface and divide the prawn mixture between them. Roll each leaf around the filling, tucking in the sides, to make a small parcel (securing with a cocktail stick if necessary).

◼ Preheat the oven to 180°C/Gas 4. Place the parcels, seam side down on a non-stick, parchment-lined baking sheet and cook for 8–10 minutes until the vegetables are just tender. Let cool completely before serving with soy and chilli sauces.

**BONUS POINT**
To make the rolling and stuffing easier, you may need to remove the tough stalks from the cabbage leaves.

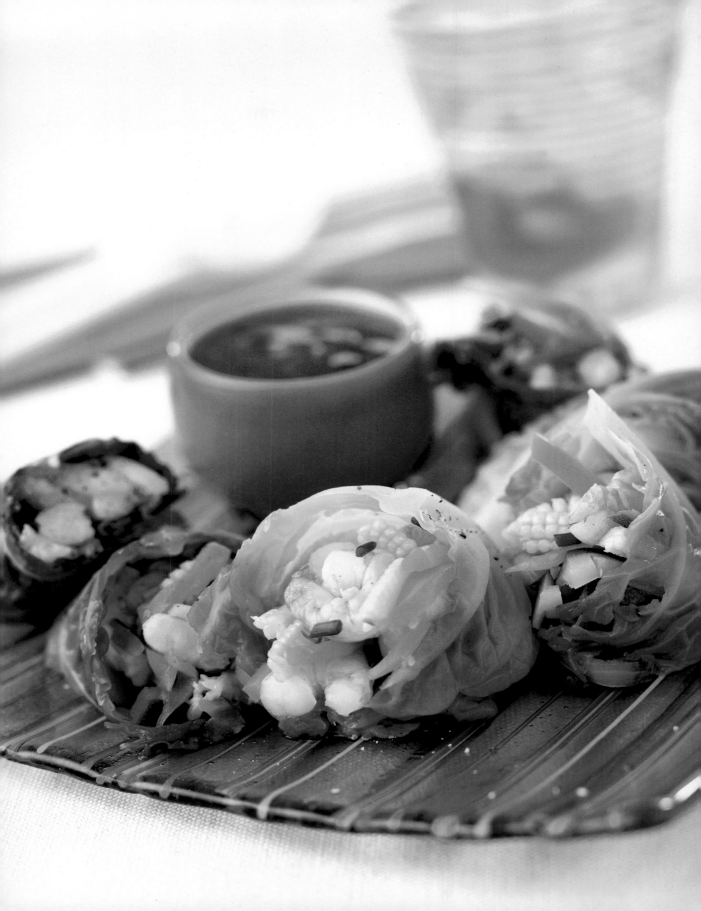

**serves** 4
**preparation time**
15 minutes
**cooking time**
8–10 minutes
**syns per serving**
original **1/2**
green **5 1/2**

# Tuna, cucumber and baby gem salad

Roasted red peppers, tuna, cucumber and crisp baby gem lettuce leaves make for a pretty and easy salad, served with a delicious fruity dressing.

**6 red peppers, deseeded**

**for the dressing:**
**juice of 1 lemon**
**100ml/3 1/2 fl oz apple juice**
**1 tsp powdered mustard**
**salt and freshly ground black pepper**

**6 spring onions, finely shredded**
**2 x 185g/6 1/2 oz cans tuna in water, drained**
**2 tbsp caperberries**
**1 cucumber, sliced thinly**
**3 plum tomatoes, cut into wedges**
**2 baby gem lettuces, leaves separated**

ORIGINAL

■ Place the red peppers skin side up under a hot grill. Cook for 8–10 minutes until charred and blistered, place in a clean plastic bag and set aside for 10 minutes.

■ Meanwhile, make the dressing by mixing together all the ingredients, season well and set aside.

■ Place the spring onions in a salad bowl. Flake in the tuna and add the caperberries, cucumber, tomatoes, gem leaves and charred red peppers. Pour over the dressing and toss to mix well. Serve at room temperature or, if desired, chill slightly before serving.

**BONUS POINT**
To lower the Syn count on a Green day, omit the tuna.

# Spicy Mexican roll

serves 4
**preparation time**
15 minutes
**syns per serving**
original **14**
green **8**

If you are watching your Syn count with these delicious spicy rolls, omit the bread and serve the chilli mix on a selection of salad leaves.

1 x 400g/14oz can red kidney beans, drained

1 chicken breast fillet, cooked and skinned

8 tbsp very low fat natural fromage frais

1 tbsp sweet chilli sauce

2 x 200g/7oz cans sweetcorn niblets, drained

4 spring onions, finely sliced

4 tbsp chopped coriander leaves

salt and freshly ground black pepper

1 red pepper, deseeded

4 x 60g/2oz wholemeal rolls

a small handful of mixed salad leaves

GREEN

■ Place the red kidney beans in a bowl and lightly mash with a fork.

■ Finely chop the chicken and stir into the beans with the fromage frais, sweet chilli sauce, sweetcorn niblets, spring onions and coriander. Add seasoning to taste.

■ Finely dice the red pepper and add to the chilli mixture.

■ Split the rolls in half and arrange the salad leaves over the bottom half. Divide the chilli mix between the four rolls and sandwich together with the top half of the rolls. Wrap in cling film and chill until needed.

**BONUS POINT**
Black-eyed beans or cannellini beans make a good alternative to the red kidney beans.

serves 4
**preparation time**
15–20 minutes
**cooking time**
50–55 minutes
**syns per serving**
original **1½**
green **9½**

ORIGINAL

# Chicken and tarragon terrine with rustic tomato sauce

On an Original day, this low Syn version of a typical chicken terrine benefits from being made more than a couple of days in advance of eating.

**600g/1lb 6oz lean chicken mince**
**2 apples, peeled, cored and roughly grated**
**4 garlic cloves, peeled and crushed**
**1 tsp smoked paprika**
**1 tbsp finely grated lemon zest**
**2 onions, peeled and very finely chopped**
**6 tbsp very finely chopped tarragon**
**salt and freshly ground black pepper**

**for the sauce:**
**1 onion, peeled and roughly diced**
**1 x 400g/14oz can chopped tomatoes**
**4 tbsp finely chopped mixed herbs (basil and parsley)**
**1 tbsp artificial sweetener**
**salt and freshly ground black pepper**

**to serve:**
**crudités, e.g. cucumber batons, celery, cherry tomatoes**

▪ Preheat the oven to 190°C/Gas 5. Line a non-stick loaf tin with non-stick baking parchment.

▪ Place the chicken mince, apples, garlic, paprika, lemon zest, onions and tarragon in a bowl. Mix thoroughly, season and spoon into the prepared loaf tin. Place in the oven and cook for 50–55 minutes or until the loaf feels firm and set and the juices run clear.

▪ Meanwhile, make the sauce by combining all the ingredients in a saucepan, bring to the boil, cover, reduce the heat and simmer gently for 15–20 minutes. Add seasoning to taste.

▪ When cool, wrap the loaf tin tightly in cling film and chill in the fridge overnight. Peel off the cling film and invert the tin onto a chopping board. Remove the tin and then the paper and cut into thick slices. Serve at room temperature with the sauce, accompanied by the crudités.

**BONUS POINT**
For a flavour change, substitute pork mince for the chicken and parsley for the tarragon.

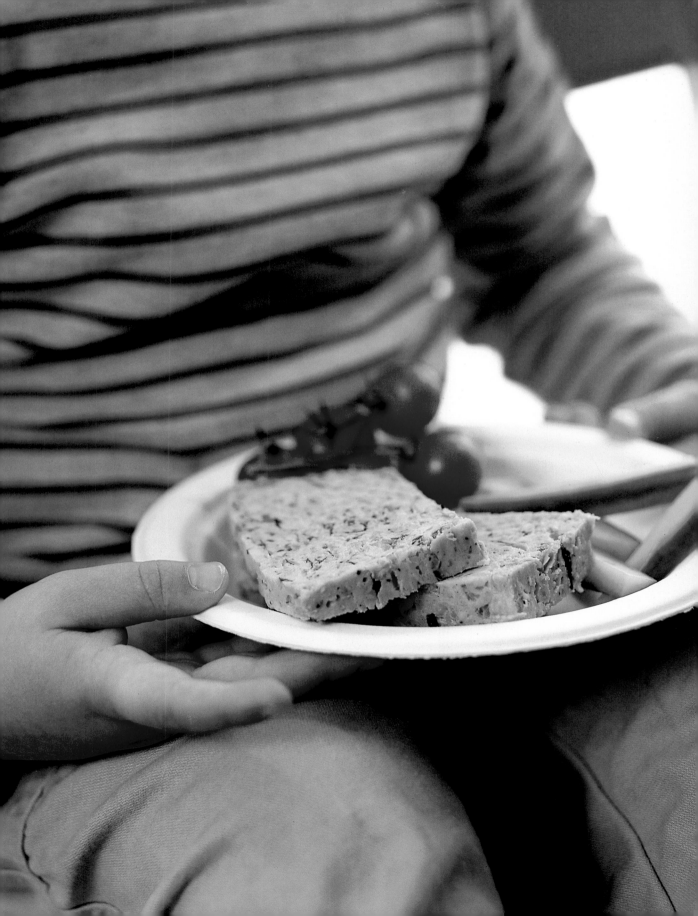

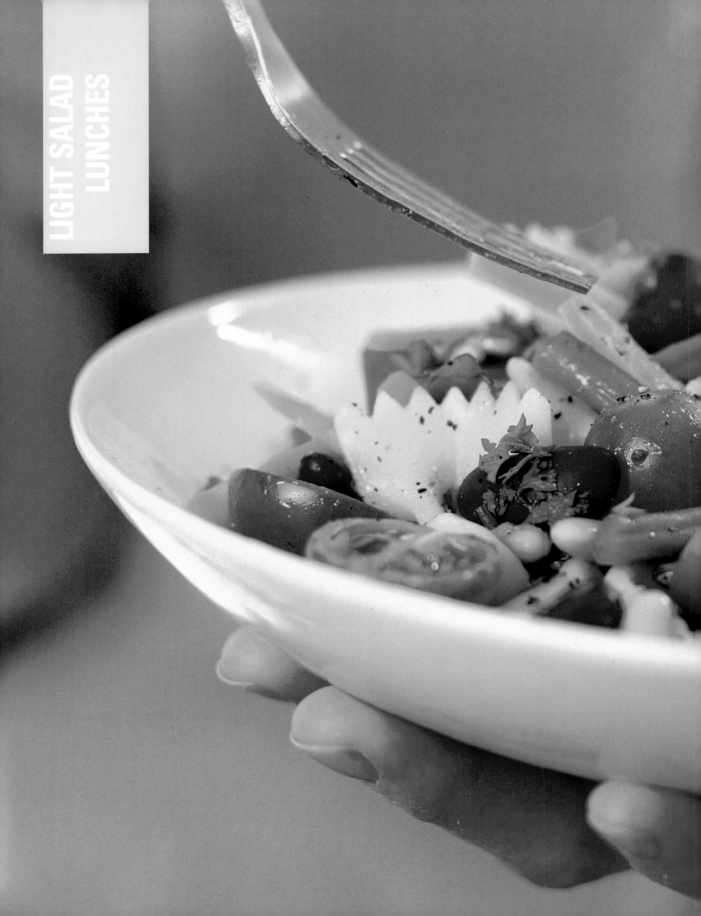

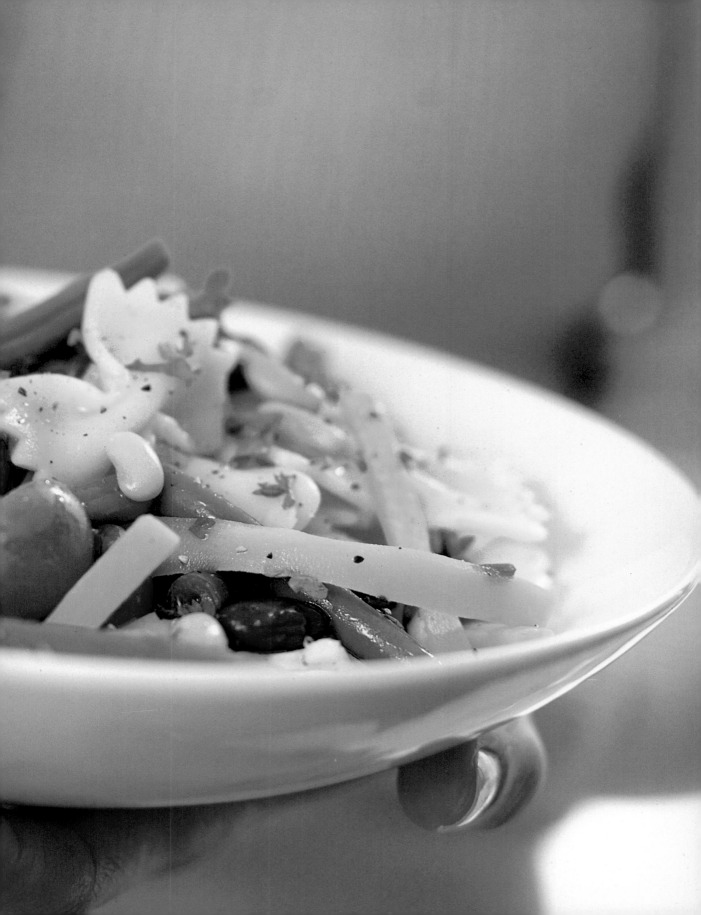

serves 4
**preparation time**
10 minutes
**cooking time**
10–12 minutes
**vegetarian**
**syns per serving**
original **1/2**
green **1/2**

# Mixed grilled pepper and basil salad

This colourful and robust salad is low in Syns on both Green and Original days and can be prepared a couple of hours ahead.

6 red peppers
6 yellow peppers

for the dressing:
1 garlic clove, peeled and crushed
3 tbsp balsamic vinegar
1 tbsp artificial sweetener

3 tbsp apple juice
salt and freshly ground black pepper

1 small red onion, peeled, halved and
   thinly sliced
a large handful of basil leaves
a small handful of wild rocket leaves

Heat the grill to hot. Halve and deseed the peppers and place skin side up on a grill rack and place under the grill for 10–12 minutes until charred and blistered. Remove and place in a clean plastic bag and set aside for 10 minutes.

Meanwhile, make the dressing by combining all the ingredients in a small bowl. Season well.

Remove the skins from the peppers and cut into thick strips. Place in a shallow salad bowl with the red onion, basil and rocket leaves. Pour over the dressing and toss to mix well. Serve at room temperature or chilled, if desired.

**BONUS POINT**
If you are in a hurry, use canned pimentos instead of the grilled peppers.

GREEN/ORIGINAL

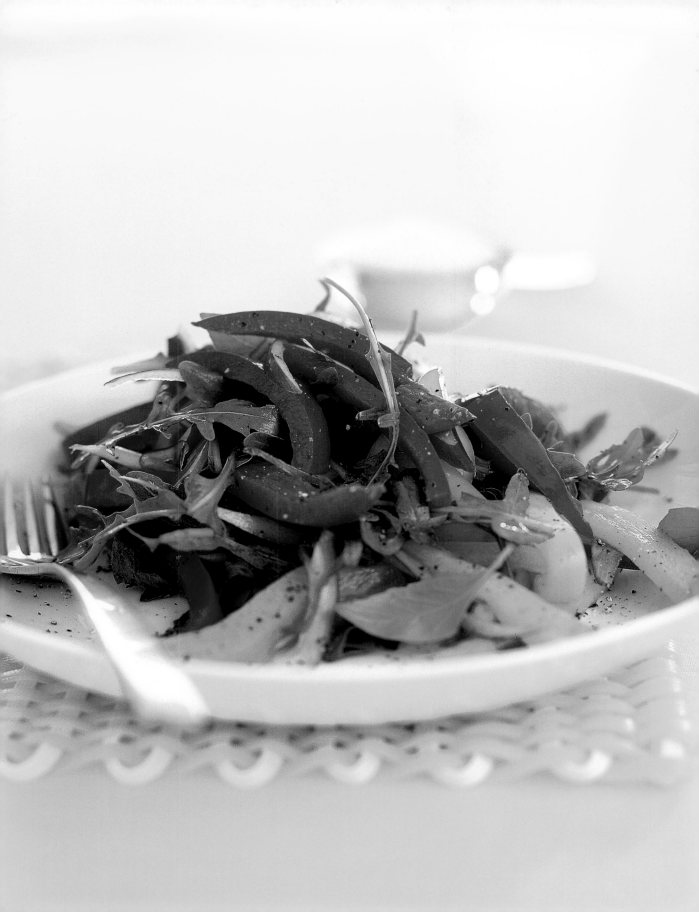

**serves** 4
**preparation time**
25 minutes
**cooking time**
about 20 minutes
**vegetarian**
**syns per serving**
original **9**
green **free**

**GREEN**

# Creamy Quorn, vegetable and pasta salad

This healthy pasta salad with its creamy, zingy dressing and crunchy vegetables makes a substantial, and yet light, lunch.

200g/7oz dried pasta shapes
200g/7oz sugar snap peas, halved
  lengthways
300g/10oz carrots, peeled and cut
  into thin batons
100g/3½oz baby sweetcorn, halved
  lengthways
1 red pepper, deseeded and cut into
  thin strips
8 spring onions, thickly sliced
200g/7oz very low fat natural
  fromage frais

200g/7oz Quark soft cheese
1 level tsp English mustard
juice and finely grated zest of 1 small
  lemon
4 tbsp freshly chopped flat-leaf
  parsley
2 tbsp chopped chives
350g/12oz Quorn pieces
salt and freshly ground black pepper

■ Cook the pasta according to the packet instructions, drain and transfer to a clean saucepan.

■ Meanwhile, cook the sugar snap peas, carrots, sweetcorn, red pepper and spring onions in a pan of rapidly boiling water for 4–5 minutes. Drain and refresh in cold water. Drain and add to the pasta.

■ Place the fromage frais, Quark, mustard, lemon juice and zest and the herbs in a food processor and blend until smooth. Pour over the pasta mixture, add the Quorn pieces and gently heat through. Season and serve at room temperature.

**BONUS POINT**
Ring the changes by using orange zest and juice in the dressing in place of the lemon.

# Ultimate celery, apple and potato salad

Boiled potatoes, sweet crunchy apples and fresh salad vegetables make great partners for the piquant mustard dressing of this delicious salad.

**serves** 4
**preparation time**
15 minutes
**vegetarian**
**syns per serving**
original **7**
green **1¹/₂**

600g/1lb 6oz baby new potatoes, scrubbed and halved
4 celery stalks, thinly sliced
4 red apples, cored and cut into bite-sized pieces
a large handful of mizuna or mixed salad leaves
6 spring onions, thinly sliced
a bunch of chives, chopped

for the dressing:
1 level tsp Dijon mustard

2 level tbsp reduced calorie mayonnaise
100g/3½oz very low fat natural fromage frais
2 tbsp chopped gherkins
salt and freshly ground black pepper

to serve:
2 hard-boiled eggs, peeled and finely chopped
chopped chives

**GREEN**

■ Boil the potatoes in lightly salted water until tender. Drain, cool and place in a large salad bowl with the celery, apples, mizuna or mixed salad leaves, spring onions and chives.

■ Make the dressing by mixing together all the ingredients in a bowl. Pour over the salad and toss to mix well.

■ To serve, scatter over the chopped egg and garnish with the chives.

**BONUS POINT**
For a slightly more grassy flavour in the salad use dill instead of chives.

**serves** 4
**preparation time**
12 minutes
**cooking time**
10 minutes
**vegetarian**
**syns per serving**
original **8**
green **free**

GREEN

# Farfalle and mixed bean salad

High in fibre, this colourful and healthy salad combines pasta, beans, carrots and tomatoes with a fruity dressing.

60g/2oz farfalle or any other pasta
  that is a short shape
350g/12oz green beans, trimmed and
  halved widthways
2 carrots, peeled and cut into thin
  matchsticks
1 x 400g/14oz can mixed beans,
  drained
100g/3½ oz cherry tomatoes, halved
4 spring onions, finely sliced

for the dressing:
4 tbsp balsamic vinegar
2 tbsp orange or pineapple juice
1–2 tbsp artificial sweetener
1–2 garlic cloves, peeled and crushed
½ tsp powdered English mustard
4 tbsp finely chopped parsley
salt and freshly ground black pepper

■ Cook the pasta according to the packet instructions, drain, refresh in cold water, drain again and place in a large bowl.

■ Blanch the green beans and carrots in a large pan of lightly salted boiling water for 2–3 minutes, drain, refresh with cold water and drain again. Add to the pasta with the mixed beans, cherry tomatoes and spring onions.

■ Make the dressing by mixing together all the ingredients, pour over the salad ingredients and toss to mix well. Season, sprinkle over the chopped herbs and serve.

**BONUS POINT**
If you are in a
rush, substitute a
fat-free French-
style dressing for
the home-made
version.

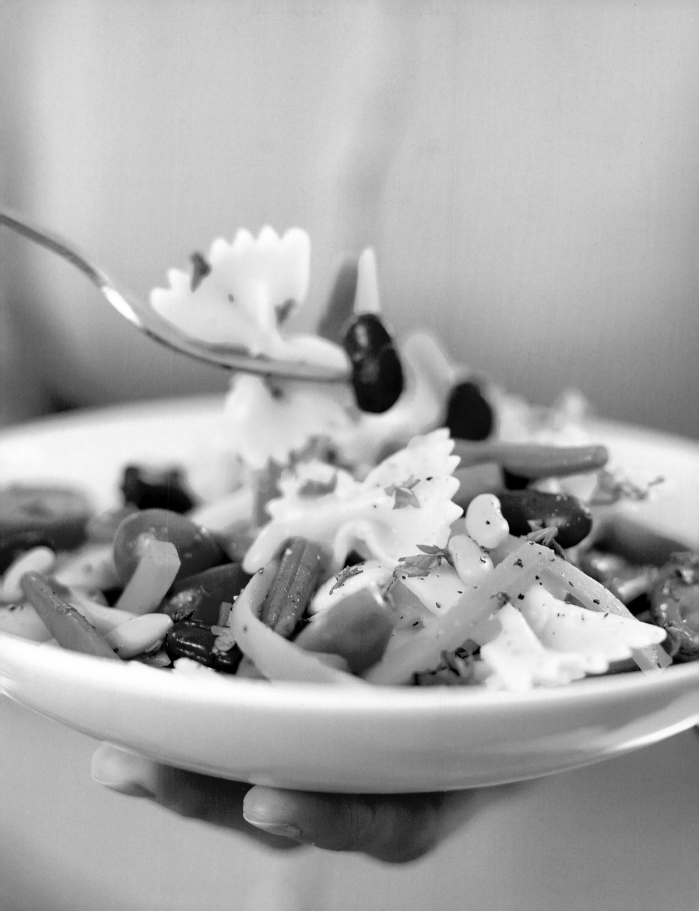

serves 4
**preparation time**
20 minutes
**vegetarian**
**syns per serving**
original 3$^1$/$_2$
green 3$^1$/$_2$

# Feta, watermelon and olive salad

Juicy pink watermelon, black grapes and red onions coupled with feta cheese and a fat-free vinaigrette make this a memorable summer salad.

$^1$/$_2$ **small, ripe watermelon**
**1 small cucumber**
$^1$/$_2$ **red onion**
**100g/3$^1$/$_2$ oz black seedless grapes**
**8 black olives**
**100g/3$^1$/$_2$ oz feta cheese**

**for the dressing:**
**6 tbsp fat-free vinaigrette dressing**
**juice of 1 lemon**
**1 tbsp chopped parsley**
**freshly ground black pepper**

Cut the skin from the watermelon with a sharp knife and cut the flesh into bite-sized pieces, discarding any seeds. Place in a large, shallow salad bowl.

Peel, halve and deseed the cucumber, slice thinly and place with the watermelon. Finely slice the red onion and add to the salad mixture, along with the grapes and the olives.

Cut the feta cheese into small cubes and scatter over the watermelon mixture.

Place all the dressing ingredients in a bowl and mix thoroughly to combine. Season and pour over the salad. Toss to mix well and serve immediately.

**BONUS POINT**
To lower your Syn count still further, omit the feta cheese.

GREEN/ORIGINAL

# North African carrot and coriander salad

This colourful and tasty salad conjures up the atmosphere of the Moroccan souks and is a terrific party piece.

500g/1lb 2oz large carrots
a large bunch of coriander leaves
juice of 1 large lemon
juice of 1 orange
$1/4$ tsp ground cumin
$1/4$ tsp ground cinnamon
salt and freshly ground black pepper

serves 4
**preparation time**
10 minutes
**cooking time**
1–2 minutes
**vegetarian**
**syns per serving**
original $1/2$
green $1/2$

■ Peel the carrots and cut them into thin matchsticks. Bring a large saucepan of lightly salted water to the boil and cook the carrots for 1–2 minutes. Drain and refresh in cold water. Drain again and place in a bowl.

■ Wash the coriander and roughly chop the leaves. Add to the carrots and toss to mix.

■ Mix together the lemon and orange juices and the ground cumin and cinnamon. Season and pour over the carrot and coriander mixture. Toss to mix well and serve at room temperature or chilled slightly, if desired.

**BONUS POINT**
This is an ideal accompaniment to grilled meat or fish.

GREEN/ORIGINAL

serves 6
**preparation time**
25 minutes
**vegetarian**
**syns per serving**
original **4¹/₂**
green **free**

# Harlequin rice salad

This tempting and vibrant salad, flavoured with dill, is colourful and full of different textures, which always looks great.

100g/3¹/₂oz cooked, cooled Basmati
  rice
1 x 100g/3½ oz can pimentos,
  drained
½ small red onion
1 x 195g/7oz can sweetcorn niblets,
  drained
1 cucumber
4 plum tomatoes
100g/3½ oz gherkins
6 tbsp chopped dill

for the dressing:
4 tbsp tarragon vinegar
2 tbsp artificial sweetener
1 level tsp Dijon mustard
1 garlic clove, crushed
salt and freshly ground black pepper

GREEN

■ Place the rice in a large bowl.

■ Finely chop the pimentos and the red onion and place in the bowl with the rice. Add the sweetcorn.

■ Halve the cucumber lengthways, deseed and chop into 1cm/¹/₂in cubes and add to the rice.

■ Finely chop the tomatoes and gherkins and add to the rice with the chopped dill.

■ For the dressing, mix together the vinegar, sweetener, mustard and garlic and add to the rice. Toss the mixture carefully to coat well, season and serve immediately.

**BONUS POINT**
Use a combination of brown Basmati and wild rice for an even more interesting-looking plateful.

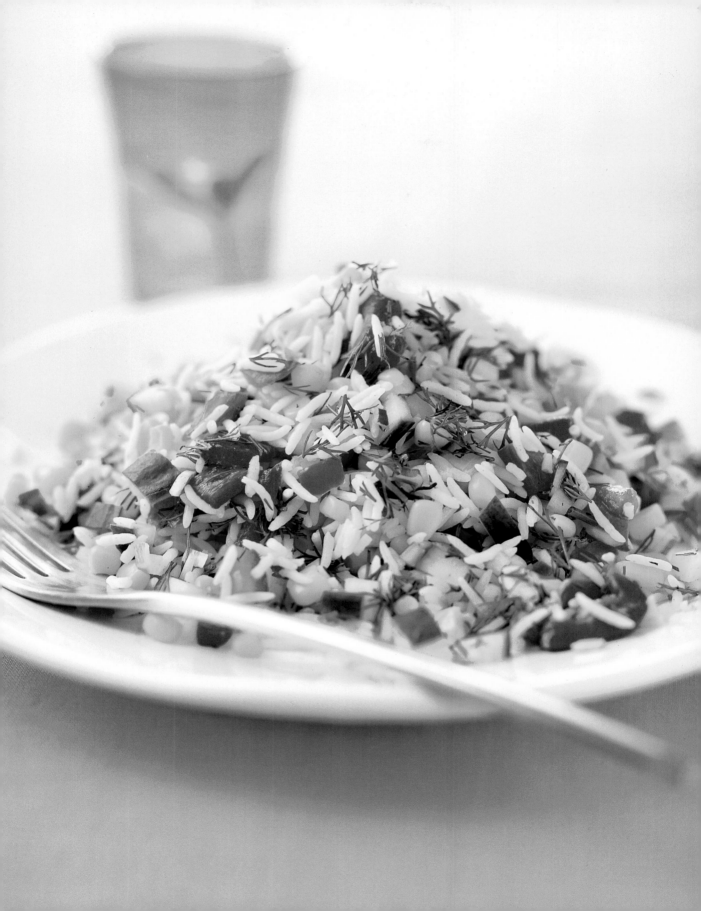

serves 4
**preparation time**
15 minutes
**cooking time**
35 minutes
**vegetarian**
**syns per serving**
original **3½**
green **free**

# Puy lentil salad

Cooked French-style lentils combined with salad vegetables and herbs make a smart, healthy and original light lunch.

100g/3½oz Puy lentils
**4 spring onions**
**15 red radishes**
**300g/10oz cherry tomatoes**
**2 celery stalks**
**a large bunch of flat-leaf parsley**
**5 tbsp fat-free French-style dressing**
**salt and freshly ground black pepper**

**to serve:**
**4 hard-boiled eggs, roughly chopped**

**GREEN**

■ Place the lentils in a large saucepan of lightly salted water and bring to the boil. Reduce the heat and cook gently for 30 minutes or until the lentils are just tender. Drain, transfer to a wide, shallow bowl and allow to cool.

■ While the lentils are cooking, finely slice the spring onions and the radishes. Cut the cherry tomatoes in half and thinly slice the celery. When the lentils are cooked, drain and add the salad vegetables.

■ Roughly chop the parsley and add to the lentil mixture. Pour over the dressing, season and toss to mix well. Sprinkle the chopped eggs over the top and serve at room temperature or slightly chilled, if desired.

**BONUS POINT**
You could cook the lentils the night before and chill in the fridge until ready to serve.

# Chilled Russian salad

Any combination of cooked diced vegetables can be used in this classic salad, which should be served chilled.

**serves** 4
**preparation time**
15 minutes
+ chilling
**cooking time**
15 minutes
**vegetarian**
**syns per serving**
original **3**
green **1½**

200g/7oz green beans
3 carrots
100g/3½ oz potatoes
100g/3½ oz fresh or frozen peas, cooked
4 cooked baby beetroot, peeled

250g/9oz very low fat natural fromage frais
1 tbsp artificial sweetener
juice of ½ lime
3 tbsp chopped flat-leaf parsley
salt and freshly ground black pepper

for the dressing:
1 level tsp Dijon mustard
2 level tbsp reduced calorie mayonnaise

to serve:
shredded iceberg lettuce leaves

■ Cut the green beans, carrots and potatoes into 1.5cm/¾in cubes. Bring two pans of lightly salted water to the boil. Add the beans and carrots to one pan and cook for 3–4 minutes. Drain and refresh in cold water. Drain and transfer to a large bowl.

■ Add the potatoes to the other saucepan and boil for 6–8 minutes or until just tender. Drain and refresh in cold water. Drain again and add to the bean and carrot mixture. Cook the peas in boiling water for 2 minutes, drain and add to this mixture.

■ Cut the beetroot into 1.5cm/¾in cubes, add to the vegetable mixture and toss to mix well.

■ Make the dressing by combining all the ingredients in a bowl and pour over the vegetables. Toss to coat evenly, season, cover and chill in the fridge for 1–2 hours. To serve, line four serving plates with shredded iceberg lettuce leaves and divide the salad on top of each serving. Serve chilled.

**GREEN**

**BONUS POINT**
This recipe is perfect for a picnic as it can be prepared the night before and served straight from the fridge.

**serves** 4
**preparation time**
15 minutes
**syns per serving**
original **1/2**
green **9 1/2**

# Prawn, mango and herb salad

Juicy pink prawns and tropical orange mangoes complement each other perfectly in this quick-to-prepare salad that makes an ideal light lunch.

ORIGINAL

**700g/1lb 9oz cooked, peeled tiger prawns**
**juice of 1 lemon or lime**
**2 ripe, juicy mangoes, peeled, stoned and roughly diced**
**a small handful of wild rocket**
**2 baby gem lettuces, trimmed and leaves separated**
**a small handful of mint leaves**

**for the dressing:**
**200g/7oz very low fat natural yogurt**
**60ml/2fl oz pineapple or mango juice**
**3–4 tbsp finely chopped dill**
**3–4 tbsp finely snipped chives**
**salt and freshly ground black pepper**

▪ Place the prawns in a large mixing bowl and pour over the lemon or lime juice. Add the mangoes, rocket, baby gem and mint leaves and toss to mix well.

▪ For the dressing, mix together the dressing ingredients and season.

▪ To serve, divide the salad between four large serving plates or bowls and drizzle the dressing over each.

**BONUS POINT**
If you have some leftover poached salmon in the fridge, cut it into cubes and use instead of the prawns.

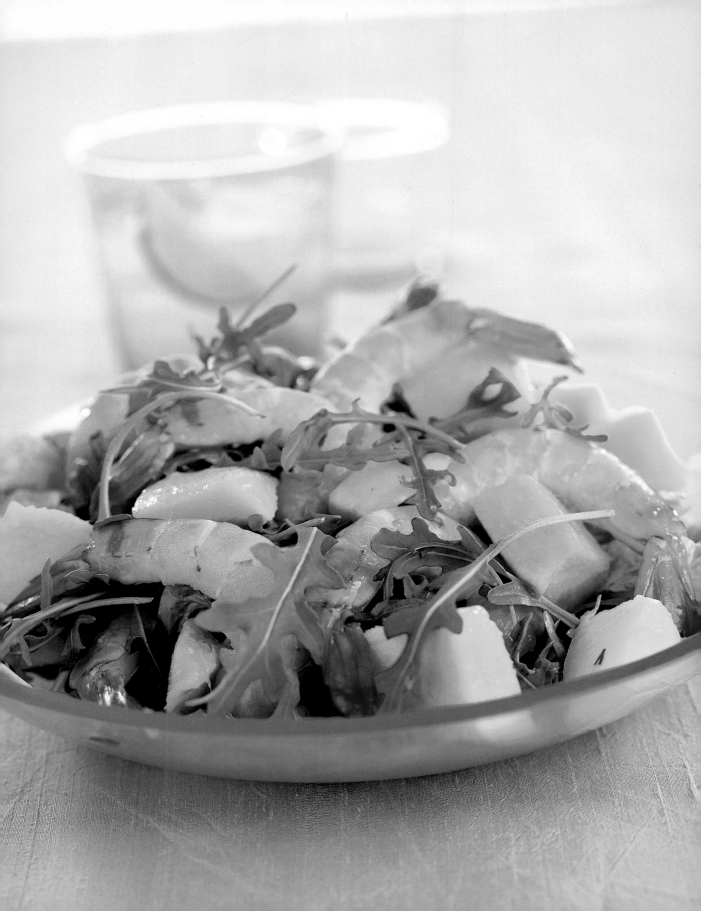

# Creamy Caesar's salad with croûtons

serves 4
**preparation time**
14 minutes
**cooking time**
6 minutes
**syns per serving**
original **3**
green **4½**

Created in 1926 by Caesar Cardini in Mexico, this classic salad is recreated here in this tasty, low-Syn version.

ORIGINAL

**for the croûtons:**
**2 thin slices day-old bread**
**1 tsp finely grated garlic**
**1 tbsp finely chopped mixed herbs**
**Fry Light for spraying**
**salt and freshly ground black pepper**

**for the dressing:**
**100ml/3½fl oz fat-free vinaigrette**
**200g/7oz very low fat natural yogurt**
**1 garlic clove, peeled and crushed**
**1 tsp powdered English mustard**
**juice of 1 lemon**

**½ tsp finely grated lemon zest**
**a few drops of Worcestershire sauce**
**1–2 drops of Tabasco sauce**
**salt and freshly ground black pepper**

**for the salad:**
**2 romaine or 1 large cos lettuce**
**60g/2oz anchovy fillets, drained**

**to serve:**
**2 level tbsp grated Parmesan cheese**
**4 hard-boiled eggs, quartered**

■ Preheat the oven to 180°C/Gas 4. Cut the bread into small cubes and place in a bowl with the garlic and herbs. Spray with Fry light, season and toss to mix well. Spray a non-stick baking sheet with Fry Light and spread the bread cubes on it in a single layer. Place in the oven for 5–6 minutes or until just turning lightly golden. Remove and set aside to cool.

■ Meanwhile, make the dressing by mixing together all the ingredients in a small bowl. Season and set aside.

■ Separate the lettuce leaves, wash and spin dry. Tear into bite-sized pieces and place in a large bowl. Roughly chop the anchovy fillets and toss with the leaves. Pour over the dressing and toss to mix well.

■ To serve, pile onto four plates and sprinkle over the grated cheese and add four wedges of boiled egg to each plate. Scatter the croûtons over the top and serve immediately.

**BONUS POINT**
Use any robust leaves instead of the romaine lettuce.

# French-style bean and tuna salad

A substantial combination of tuna, mixed leaves, mixed beans, tomatoes and eggs, this makes a great lunch special.

**serves** 4
**preparation time**
15 minutes
**cooking time**
2–3 minutes
**syns per serving**
original **7**
green **5**

100g/3½ oz green beans, trimmed and halved widthways

1 large red onion, peeled, halved and very thinly sliced

100g/3½ oz mixed salad leaves

1 x 400g/14oz can cannellini beans, drained

1 x 200g/7oz can sweetcorn niblets, drained

1 cucumber, halved and thinly sliced

4 ripe plum tomatoes, cut into wedges

for the dressing:

2 tbsp fat-free French-style dressing

1 garlic clove, peeled and crushed

1 tbsp very finely chopped dill

1 tsp very finely grated lemon zest

juice of 1 lemon

salt and freshly ground black pepper

2 x 185g/6½ oz cans tuna in water, drained

6 eggs (boiled to your liking and halved)

GREEN

■ Blanch the beans in a large pan of lightly salted boiling water for 2–3 minutes. Then drain and place in a wide, shallow bowl with the red onion, mixed salad leaves, cannellini beans, sweetcorn, cucumber and tomatoes.

■ Mix the French-style dressing with the garlic, chopped dill and lemon zest and juice, season and set aside.

■ Divide the salad between four large serving plates. Flake the tuna into large pieces, scatter over the salad and arrange three boiled egg halves on each plate. Drizzle dressing over each salad and serve immediately.

**BONUS POINT**
For a vegetarian option, omit the tuna and replace with boiled new potatoes, which are Free Food on a Green day.

**ORIGINAL**

**serves** 4
**preparation time**
20 minutes
**syns per serving**
original **½**
green **8**

# Fruity chicken salad with a creamy tarragon and mustard dressing

A tasty salad of cooked chicken, which is tossed together with sweet, crisp grapes and other salad vegetables in a creamy, herbed dressing.

4 cooked chicken breast fillets, skinned and cut into bite-sized pieces
200g/7oz green seedless grapes, halved
1 large cucumber, skinned, deseeded and roughly chopped
1 red and 1 yellow pepper, deseeded and cut into strips

for the dressing:
200g/7oz very low fat natural yogurt
juice of 1 lemon
60ml/2fl oz pineapple juice
2 level tsp wholegrain mustard
2 tbsp finely chopped tarragon
salt and freshly ground black pepper
a large handful of mixed salad leaves

◻ Place the chicken into a large, shallow bowl with the grapes and cucumber.

◻ Heat a griddle pan on high, place the strips of pepper on it and cook for 4–5 minutes until just tender. Transfer to the chicken and fruit mixture.

◻ For the dressing, place the yogurt and the lemon and pineapple juices in a bowl and whisk until smooth. Stir in the mustard and tarragon. Season and pour over the chicken mixture. Toss to mix well.

◻ To serve, divide the mixed salad leaves between four shallow bowls or plates. Top with the chicken salad and serve immediately.

**BONUS POINT**
For something a bit spicier, use store bought spicy chicken (skinless) instead of the plain cooked chicken.

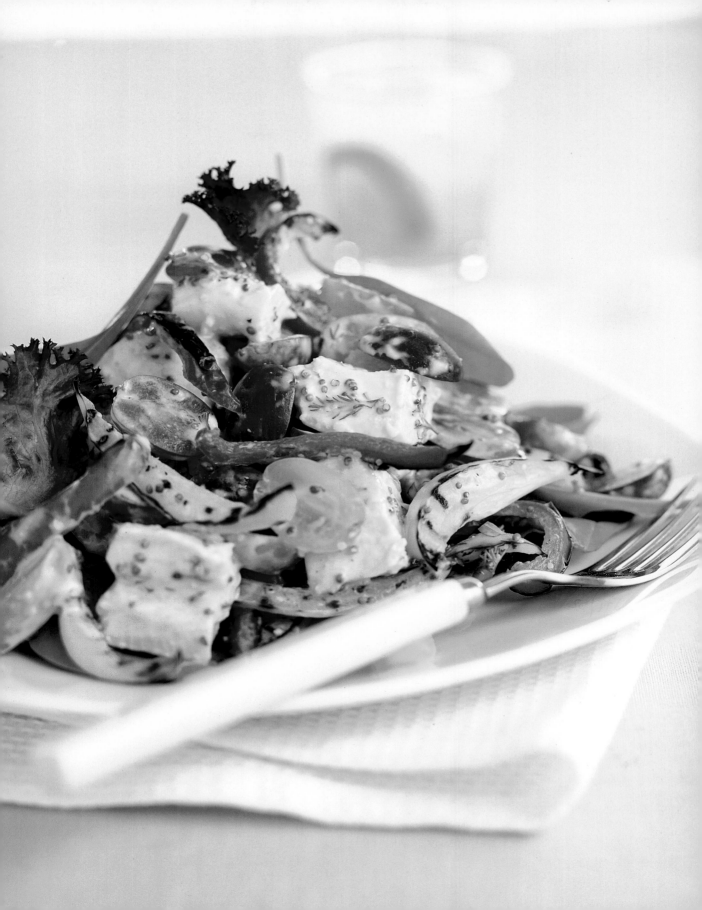

ORIGINAL

**serves** 4
**preparation time**
15–20 minutes +
4–5 hours
marinating
**cooking time**
6–8 minutes
**syns per serving**
original **free**
green **10½**

# Warm spiced chicken and spinach salad

In this salad, East meets West with the oriental spices and flavours of the chicken and dressing combined with a very western-style dish.

800g/1lb 12oz mini chicken breast
   fillets
1 tbsp finely grated lemon zest
juice of 2 lemons
2 tsp finely grated garlic
2 tsp finely grated ginger
3 tbsp mild or medium curry powder
salt
100g/3½ oz baby leaf spinach
3 plum tomatoes, quartered

**for the dressing:**
200g/7oz very low fat natural yogurt
2 tbsp very finely chopped mint
   leaves
2 tbsp very finely chopped coriander
   leaves
salt
Fry Light for spraying

**to serve:**
paprika to sprinkle (optional)
lime or lemon wedges

■ Place the chicken in a mixing bowl. Mix together the lemon zest and juice, garlic, ginger and curry powder. Season with salt and pour over the chicken. Toss to mix well and then cover and marinate in the fridge for 4–5 hours, or overnight if time permits.

■ Divide the spinach leaves and tomato wedges between four serving plates.

■ For the dressing, mix together the yogurt, mint and coriander in a small bowl. Season with salt and set aside.

**BONUS POINT**
This salad can be served cold or at room temperature. Cook the chicken in advance and chill until you are ready to use it.

■ Heat a large, non-stick frying pan until hot and spray with Fry Light. Add the chicken mixture and stir-fry over a medium heat for 6–8 minutes or until the chicken is cooked through. Divide the mixture between the four prepared plates and drizzle over the yogurt dressing. Sprinkle with paprika (if desired) and serve immediately with wedges of lime or lemon.

# Spicy Thai-style beef salad

Fragrant and aromatic with Far Eastern herbs and sauces, this is a substantial salad of beef with crisp and crunchy vegetables.

serves 4
**preparation time**
15 minutes
+ 4–5 hours
marinating time
**cooking time**
8–10 minutes
**syns per serving**
original **free**
green **8**

**450g/1lb thick beef fillet steaks (all visible fat removed)**

**for the marinade:**
4 tbsp light soy sauce
2 garlic cloves, peeled and crushed
4 tbsp finely chopped lemongrass
1 tbsp artificial sweetener
1–2 chillies, deseeded and finely chopped
1 tsp finely grated ginger
1 tsp finely grated lime zest
juice of 3 limes

**for the salad:**
1 carrot, peeled and grated

4 baby gem lettuces, trimmed and washed
1 small cucumber, deseeded and thinly sliced
60g/2oz beansprouts
4 spring onions, finely shredded
4 tbsp roughly chopped coriander leaves
2 tbsp chopped mint leaves

**for the dressing:**
3 tbsp soy sauce
1 tbsp sweet chilli sauce
juice of 2 limes
1 tbsp artificial sweetener
salt and freshly ground black pepper

■ Place the steaks in shallow mixing bowl. Mix together the marinade ingredients and pour this over the steaks. Cover and leave to marinate for a few hours (but preferably overnight) in the fridge.

■ Place all the salad ingredients in a large bowl. In a separate, smaller, bowl, mix together all the dressing ingredients and season. Pour over the salad and toss.

■ Preheat the grill to hot and then remove the steaks from the marinade. Place on a grill rack under the grill and cook for 4–5 minutes on each side, or until cooked to your liking. Remove, cover and let rest for 5 minutes before cutting into very thin slices. Divide the salad mixture between four plates, top with the beef steaks and serve immediately.

**BONUS POINT**
For a vegetarian option, omit the beef and increase the raw vegetable content.

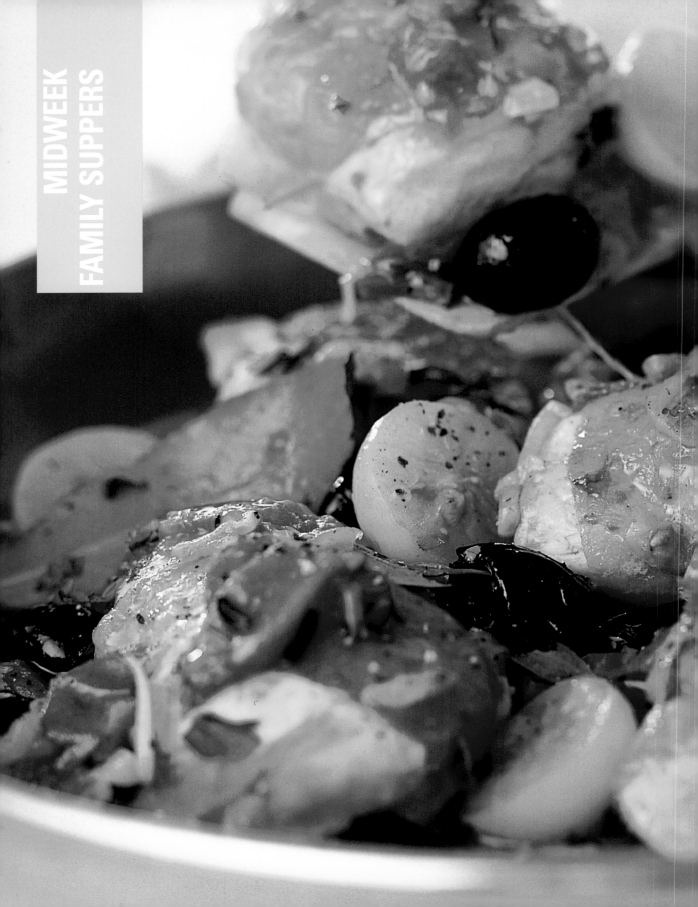

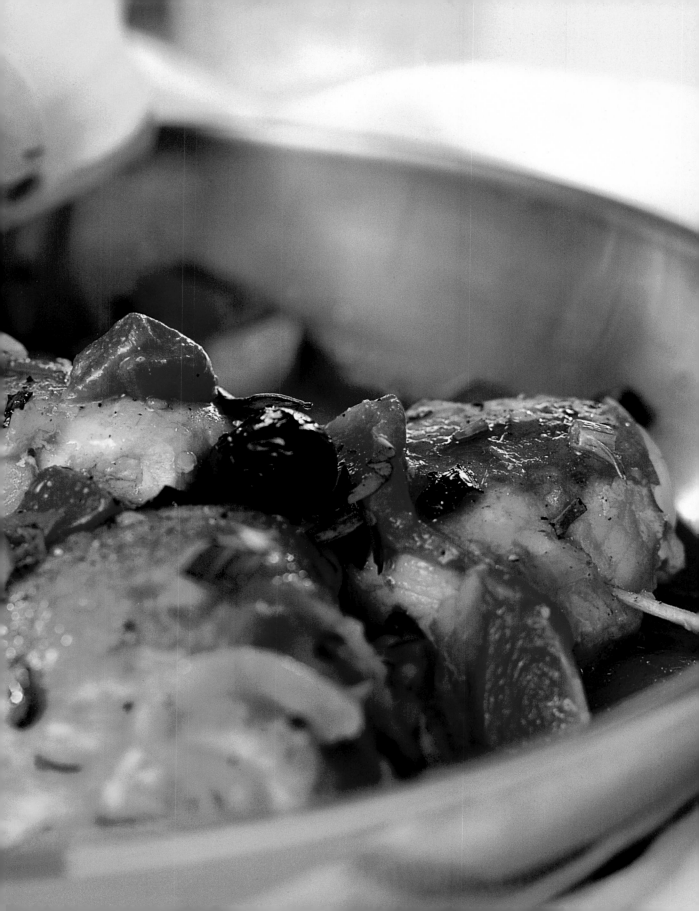

**serves** 4
**preparation time**
10 minutes
**cooking time**
about 25 minutes
+ 10 minutes
standing time
**vegetarian**
**syns per serving**
original **18½**
green **free**

GREEN

# Fragrant carrot, pea and tomato pilaff

This tasty, aromatic rice and vegetable dish makes a simple-to-prepare meal. It is perfect accompanied with a chopped cucumber salad.

Fry Light for spraying
2 onions, peeled, halved and thinly sliced
1 tsp finely grated ginger
1 tsp finely grated or crushed garlic
2 tsp ground cumin
1 tsp ground coriander
1 bay leaf
3 cloves
3 cardamom pods
2 carrots, peeled and diced

1 x 400g/14oz can chopped tomatoes
400g/14oz easy-cook Basmati rice
650ml/1pt 2fl oz boiling hot water
salt
100g/3½oz peas

to serve:
chopped coriander leaves
chopped red onion

■ Spray a large, non-stick saucepan with Fry Light. Add the onions and cook over a medium heat for 5–6 minutes until softened.

■ Add the ginger, garlic, cumin, coriander, bay leaf, cloves and cardamom pods. Stir-fry for 2–3 minutes and then add the carrots, chopped tomatoes, rice and water or stock. Season, bring back to the boil, cover tightly and cook on low for 12–15 minutes.

■ Stir in the peas and then cover and cook for a further 2–3 minutes until the rice is tender and moist. Remove from the heat and let stand for 10 minutes before fluffing up the grains with a fork. Garnish with chopped coriander leaves and serve immediately with chopped red onion.

**BONUS POINT**
This dish can be frozen up to three weeks in advance. Defrost thoroughly and heat, covered, in a medium oven for 25 minutes or until piping hot.

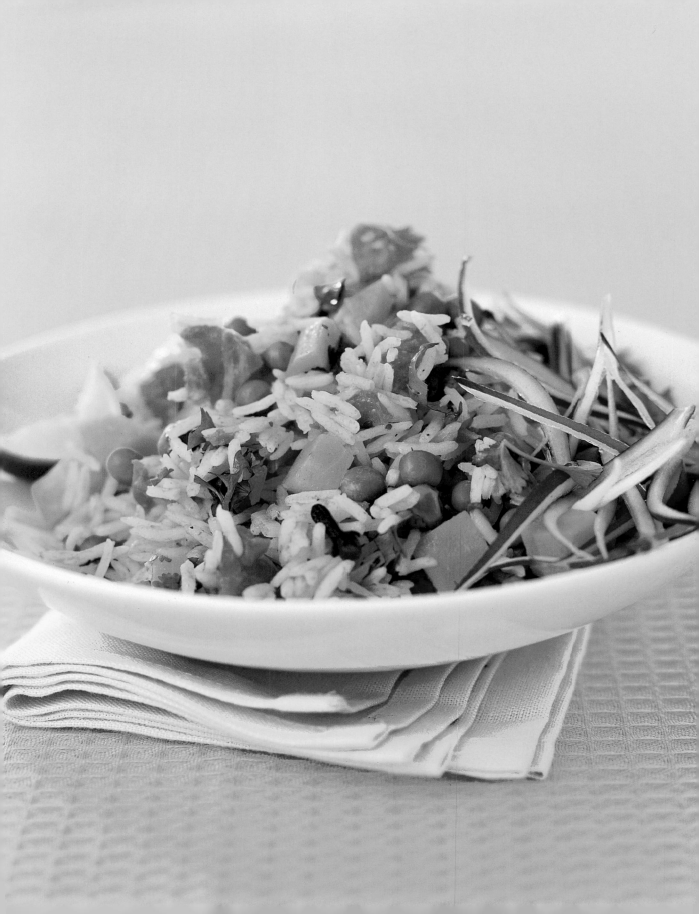

serves 4
**preparation time**
15 minutes
**cooking time**
20–25 minutes
**vegetarian**
**syns per serving**
original **6½**
green **½**

# Spinach and courgette cannelloni

This classic Italian-style comfort food combines all the colours of the nation's flag in this perfect family supper.

1 large courgette
250g/9oz baby leaf spinach
150g/5oz Quark soft cheese
150g/5oz very low fat natural
   cottage cheese
4 garlic cloves, peeled and crushed
1 red chilli, deseeded and finely
   chopped
3 tbsp chopped mint leaves
3 tbsp chopped flat-leaf parsley

1 egg yolk
salt and freshly ground black pepper
12 cannelloni tubes
Fry Light for spraying
600ml/1pt passata with herbs
2 tbsp artificial sweetener
1 level tbsp grated Parmesan cheese

to serve:
basil leaves

**GREEN**

■ Preheat the oven to 200°C/Gas 6. Cut the courgette into 1cm/½in cubes and roughly chop the spinach. Bring a large saucepan of water to the boil and blanch the courgette and spinach for 30 seconds. Drain and place in a mixing bowl.

■ In a separate bowl, mix together the Quark, cottage cheese, garlic, chilli, mint, parsley and egg yolk. Add the mixture to the courgette and spinach mixture, season and mix well.

■ Spoon the mixture into the cannelloni tubes and place in a single layer in an ovenproof dish (sprayed with Fry Light) to fit snugly. Mix together the passata and sweetener, season well and pour over the stuffed cannelloni tubes. Sprinkle over the cheese and bake for 20–25 minutes until bubbling and cooked through.

■ Serve on warmed plates, garnished with basil leaves accompanied by a crisp green salad.

**BONUS POINT**
This dish can be frozen for up to three weeks after being cooked. Defrost and heat thoroughly before serving.

# Special macaroni cheese

A special family meal based on the old favourite, this grown-up pasta dish makes for a great midweek supper.

**serves** 4
**preparation time**
20 minutes
**cooking time**
about 30 minutes
**vegetarian**
**syns per serving**
original **24**
green **6½**

400g/14oz macaroni or any other
  short-shaped pasta
Fry Light for spraying
1 small onion, peeled and very finely
  chopped
2 garlic cloves, peeled and crushed
200g/7oz closed cap mushrooms,
  quartered
8 baby leeks, thinly sliced
400g/14oz small plum tomatoes,
  roughly chopped
salt and freshly ground black pepper

for the topping:
2 level tbsp cornflour
1 level tsp Dijon mustard
300ml/½pt skimmed milk
200g/7oz very low fat natural yogurt
2 tsp garlic salt
100g/3½oz reduced-fat Cheddar
  cheese, coarsely grated
a pinch of grated nutmeg
salt and freshly ground black pepper

to garnish:
chopped parsley (optional)

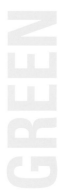

GREEN

■ Cook the macaroni according to the packet instructions, drain and set aside. Spray a large, non-stick frying pan with Fry Light and cook the onion, garlic, mushrooms and leeks over a high heat for 2–3 minutes. Add 60ml/2fl oz water to the pan, reduce the heat and cook gently for 8–10 minutes until the leeks have softened. Stir in the tomatoes, remove from the heat and mix with the drained pasta. Season well and place in a medium-sized ovenproof dish. Preheat the oven to 180°C/Gas 4.

■ Make the topping by blending the cornflour and mustard with 4 table-spoons of the milk until smooth. Heat the remaining milk in a saucepan and bring to the boil, reduce the heat and stir in the cornflour mixture and cook for 2–3 minutes until thickened. Remove from the heat and stir in the yogurt, garlic salt, cheese and nutmeg. Season well and pour over the pasta mixture. Bake in the oven for 25–30 minutes until lightly browned. Serve immediately, garnished with chopped parsley, if desired, and accompanied by a lightly dressed green salad.

**BONUS POINT**
To boost your fibre intake, use wholemeal pasta.

**serves** 4
**preparation time**
15 minutes
**cooking time**
1 hour
**vegetarian**
**syns per serving**
original **9**
green **3**

**GREEN**

# Roasted vegetable lasagne

Lasagne is a real family favourite and this recipe with a twist (roasted vegetables) will go down a treat.

2 aubergines, cut into bite-sized
   pieces
2 courgettes, cut into bite-sized
   pieces
2 red peppers, deseeded and cut into
   bite-sized pieces
2 red onions, peeled and cut into
   bite-sized pieces
6 sprigs of thyme
salt and freshly ground black pepper
Fry Light for spraying
2 level tbsp cornflour

$1/4$ tsp ground nutmeg
$1/2$ tsp ground mixed spice
190ml/7fl oz skimmed milk
200g/7oz very low fat natural
   yogurt
1 x 400g/14oz can chopped tomatoes
200ml/7fl oz passata
2 tbsp finely chopped rosemary
2 tsp finely grated garlic
10 pre-cooked lasagne sheets
1 level tbsp grated Parmesan cheese

■ Preheat the oven to 200°C/Gas 6. Place the vegetable pieces on two large, non-stick baking sheets. Scatter over the thyme sprigs, and seasoning and spray lightly with Fry Light. Roast in the oven for 15–20 minutes or until the vegetables are just tender.

■ Make a paste with the cornflour, nutmeg, mixed spice and 3–4 tbsp of the milk. In a small saucepan, bring the remaining milk to the boil and stir in the cornflour mixture. Stir and cook for 1–2 minutes until thickened, remove from the heat and stir in the yogurt. Season and set aside.

■ Remove the vegetables from the oven and transfer to a mixing bowl. Stir in the tomatoes, passata, rosemary and garlic, add seasoning and spoon half the mixture into a medium-sized ovenproof dish. Cover with half the lasagne sheets and half the yogurt sauce. Layer the rest of the vegetables on top and cover with the remaining lasagne sheets and the sauce. Sprinkle over the cheese and bake for 45 minutes or until lightly browned. Serve with a crisp green salad.

**BONUS POINT**
To save $1/2$ a Syn per serving, omit the Parmesan cheese.

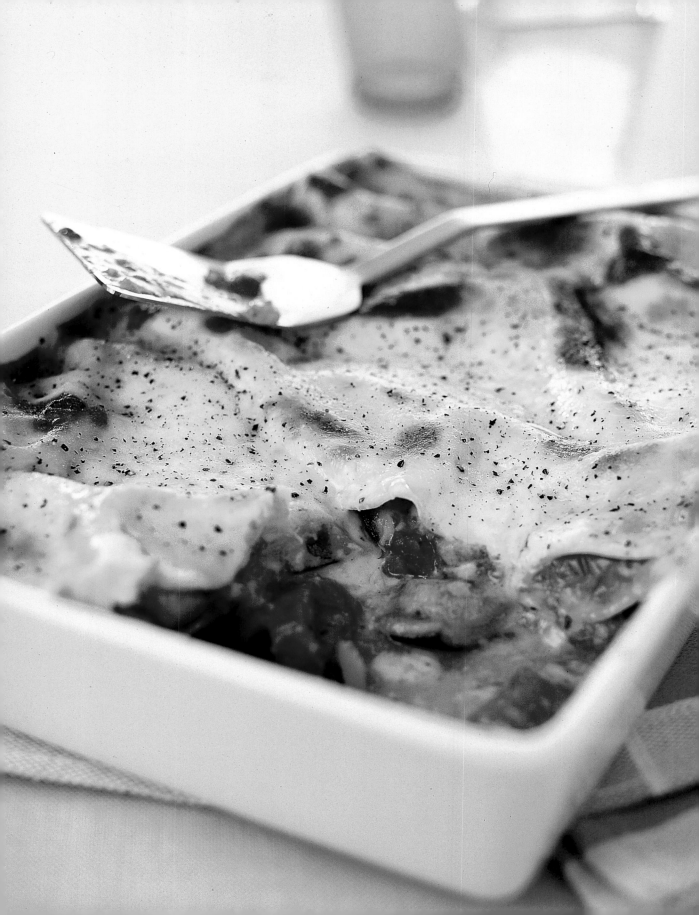

**serves** 4
**preparation time**
15 minutes
**cooking time**
about 45 minutes
**vegetarian**
**syns per serving**
original **23**
green **1/2**

GREEN

# Spaghetti Bolognese

Completely delicious and totally Free on a Green day (if you foresake the Parmesan cheese), this is a truly hearty pasta dish.

**For the Bolognese sauce:**
**Fry Light for spraying**
**1 large red onion, peeled and finely**
   **chopped**
**3 garlic cloves, thinly sliced**
**3 celery sticks, finely chopped**
**3 carrots, peeled and finely chopped**
**1 tsp chopped rosemary leaves**
**1 bay leaf**
**350g/12oz Quorn mince**
**2 x 400g/14oz cans chopped**
   **tomatoes**

**4 tbsp chopped basil leaves**
**1 tsp dried mixed herbs**
**$1/4$–$1/2$ tsp chilli flakes**
**2 tbsp artificial sweetener**
**salt and freshly ground black pepper**

**1 x 500g/1lb 2oz packet dried**
   **spaghetti**
**1 level tbsp grated Parmesan cheese**

**to garnish:**
**basil leaves**

■ Spray a large, non-stick saucepan with Fry Light and place over a medium heat. Add the onion, garlic, celery, carrots and the rosemary and bay leaf and stir-fry for 2–3 minutes. Add the Quorn mince and stir-fry for another 3–4 minutes.

■ Add the tomatoes, basil, mixed herbs, chilli flakes and the sweetener and bring to the boil, stirring often. Reduce the heat, cover and simmer gently for 35–40 minutes (stirring occasionally) until thickened. Season.

■ Meanwhile, cook the spaghetti according to the packet instructions, drain and divide between four large, warmed serving plates or shallow bowls. Top with the Bolognese sauce and sprinkle with the grated cheese, if using. Garnish each serving with basil leaves and serve immediately.

**BONUS POINT**
You could use the sauce with any pasta shape, or with rice.

# Mild and creamy Quorn curry

Forget the unhealthy midweek curry take-away and try this delicious option for a special family supper.

**serves** 4
**preparation time**
20 minutes
**cooking time**
about 30 minutes
**vegetarian**
**syns per serving**
original **free**
green **free**

1 onion, peeled and finely chopped
1 garlic clove, peeled and crushed
350g/12oz Quorn pieces
2 tbsp mild curry powder
2 carrots, peeled and cut into bite-sized pieces
1 large courgette, cut into bite-sized pieces
1 red pepper, deseeded and cut into bite-sized pieces

200g/7oz shiitake mushrooms, halved
1 x 400g/14oz can chopped tomatoes
150ml/¼pt water
salt and freshly ground black pepper
200g/7oz very low fat natural yogurt

to garnish:
chopped coriander leaves
lime wedges

■ Place the onion and garlic in a large, non-stick saucepan and cook over a gentle heat for 3–4 minutes, stirring often. Add the Quorn pieces, curry powder, the vegetables and the chopped tomatoes together with the water or stock and bring to the boil.

■ Cover the pan, reduce the heat to low and gently cook for 20–25 minutes until the vegetables are tender, stirring occasionally. Season to taste.

■ To serve, stir the yogurt until smooth and stir into the curry. Garnish with chopped coriander leaves and lime wedges.

**FREE FOOD**

**BONUS POINT**
You can vary this dish by using different vegetables as an alternative to the carrots, courgettes and mushrooms.

**serves** 6
**preparation time**
25 minutes
**cooking time**
30 minutes
**syns per serving**
original **9**
green **1**

GREEN

# Piquant vegetable cottage pie

This ultimate comfort food dish is given a low-fat twist but is packed with all the flavour of the real thing.

**for the topping:**
**900g/2lb potatoes, peeled and**
  **roughly chopped**
**4 tbsp very low fat natural yogurt**
**a pinch of grated nutmeg**
**1/2 tsp ground cinnamon**
**1/2 tsp cayenne pepper**
**salt and freshly ground black pepper**

**for the pie:**
**2 red onions, peeled and finely**
  **chopped**
**3 carrots, peeled and diced**

**2 red peppers, deseeded and diced**
**2 tsp finely grated or crushed garlic**
**1/2 tsp dried red chilli flakes**
**350g/12oz Quorn mince**
**1 level tbsp cornflour mixed with**
  **2 tbsp cold water**
**400ml/14fl oz beef stock made from**
  **Bovril**
**3 tbsp chopped flat-leaf parsley**
**1 tbsp very finely chopped rosemary**
  **leaves**
**1 egg, lightly beaten**

■ Place the potatoes in a large pan of boiling, lightly salted water and boil for 10–12 minutes or until tender. Drain, return to the pan and mash until smooth, adding the yogurt, nutmeg, cinnamon, cayenne pepper and seasoning. Set aside.

■ Preheat the oven to 200°C/Gas 6. Place all the pie ingredients except the egg in a large saucepan and bring to the boil. Reduce the heat and cover and cook gently for 5 minutes.

■ Transfer the Quorn mixture into a medium-sized ovenproof dish. Spoon over the potato mixture to cover and lightly swirl with a fork. Brush the egg over the top and bake in the oven for 25–30 minutes or until the top is lightly golden. Serve immediately with a crisp green salad.

**BONUS POINT**
The cottage pie can be frozen for up to three weeks. Defrost and heat thoroughly before serving.

# Fish and 'chips' with 'tartar' sauce

The old family favourite has been given a makeover here, with parsnip 'chips' replacing the potato ones in this healthy and delicious supper.

**serves** 4
**preparation time**
25 minutes
**cooking time**
14–18 minutes
**syns per serving**
original **10**
green **8**

**for the 'chips':**
**1 kg/2lb 4oz large parsnips, peeled and cut into thick 'fingers'**
**sea salt and freshly ground black pepper**

**for the fish:**
**finely grated zest and juice of 1 lemon**
**2 tsp garlic salt**
**4 x 200g/7oz thick cod fillets, skinned**

**for the 'tartar' sauce:**
**200g/7oz very low fat natural fromage frais**
**4 tbsp chopped dill**
**1 small cucumber, very finely chopped**
**1 small red onion, peeled and very finely chopped**

**breadcrumbs made from 2 slices of Nimble wholemeal bread**
**2 eggs, lightly beaten**

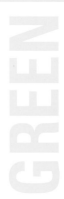

**GREEN**

■ Bring a large pan of lightly salted water to the boil and cook the parsnips for 2–3 minutes. Drain and dry on kitchen paper.

■ Preheat the oven to 200°C/Gas 6. Mix together the lemon zest, juice and garlic salt and season with black pepper. Place the cod fillets in a shallow mixing bowl and pour the mixture over them. Set aside. For the 'tartar' sauce, mix together all the ingredients in a bowl, season and chill.

■ Place the breadcrumbs on a plate and the beaten eggs in a shallow bowl. Dip each fillet into the egg and then into the breadcrumbs to coat evenly. Spray two non-stick baking sheets with Fry Light and place the fish on one of them. Spread out the parsnips on the other, season and spray with Fry Light. Place both sheets in the oven and cook for 12–15 minutes until the fish is cooked through and the parsnips tender and lightly browned. Serve immediately with the tartar sauce on the side.

**BONUS POINT**
Use any thick, firm fish fillet such as salmon, haddock or halibut as a substitute for the cod.

**serves** 4
**preparation time**
20 minutes
**cooking time**
1 hour
**syns per serving**
original **½**
green **10**

# Provençal pan-cooked chicken

This easy-to-prepare, French-style dish, bursting with flavours from Provence, is sure to become one of the family's favourite supper dishes.

Fry Light for spraying
2 large onions, peeled, halved and sliced
4 garlic cloves, peeled and thinly sliced
600ml/1pt chicken stock made from Bovril
3–4 small preserved lemons, roughly chopped
4 chicken breast fillets, skinned
4 lean bacon rashers (rind removed and cut in half)

4 ripe plum tomatoes, roughly chopped
a small bunch of tarragon, roughly chopped
1 bay leaf
10 black olives
1 x 400g/14oz can pimentos in brine, drained
salt and freshly ground black pepper

to serve:
chopped flat-leaf parsley

■ Spray a large, deep, non-stick frying pan with Fry Light and place over a medium heat. Add the onions and stir-fry for 5–6 minutes until slightly softened. Add the garlic and the stock and bring to the boil. Cook rapidly for 10 minutes, stir in the preserved lemons and then cover and simmer gently for 10–15 minutes.

■ Meanwhile, cut each chicken breast in half widthways, and wrap with half a bacon rasher, securing with a cocktail stick. Add to the pan with the tomatoes, tarragon and bay leaf, cover the pan and cook gently for 25–30 minutes or until the chicken is tender and the sauce reduced and thickened.

■ Stir in the olives, roughly chop the pimentos, add to the chicken and cook gently for 4–5 minutes. Season well and serve garnished with chopped parsley and accompanied by carrots and broccoli.

**BONUS POINT**
For a better flavour, try using organic or free-range chicken.

116

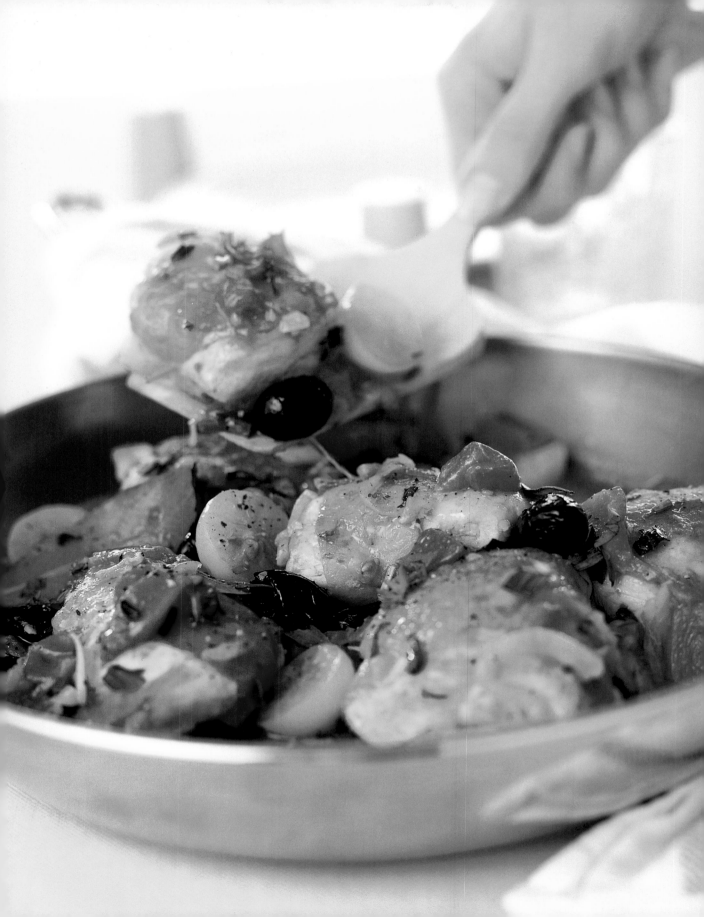

**serves** 4
**preparation time**
20 minutes
**cooking time**
20–25 minutes
**syns per serving**
original **2**
green **9½**

# Herb and garlic chicken Kievs

Great for a midweek supper, once prepared and placed in the oven you can relax until they are ready to serve.

**4 large chicken breasts, skinned and boned**
**salt and freshly ground black pepper**
**60g/2oz Quark soft cheese**
**1 garlic clove, peeled and crushed**
**1 tbsp very finely chopped parsley**
**1 tbsp very finely chopped taragon**
**4 slices Nimble wholemeal bread**
**3 eggs**
**Fry Light for spraying**

**to serve:**
**green vegetables**

Place the chicken breasts on a work surface and, using a small, sharp knife, make two slits in each breast lengthways, to create a 'pocket'. Season the breasts and set aside.

Mix together the Quark soft cheese, garlic and chopped herbs. Season well and, using a small spoon, stuff the mixture into the chicken 'pockets'.

Place the bread in a food processor and chop to make coarse bread-crumbs. Transfer to a shallow bowl.

Preheat the oven to 200°C/Gas 6.

**BONUS POINT**
These Kievs can be prepared a few hours in advance. Cover and chill them in the fridge before cooking.

In another shallow bowl, lightly beat the eggs with 1 tbsp water. Dip the chicken breasts into the egg and then roll in the breadcrumbs to coat evenly. Place on a non-stick baking sheet, spray with Fry Light and bake in the oven for 20–25 minutes until golden and cooked through. Serve the chicken Kievs with a selection of green vegetables.

# Pork and apple stew with swede mash

The flavours of pork and sweet apple make perfect partners in this warming family casserole.

**serves** 4
**preparation time**
15 minutes
**cooking time**
45–50 minutes
**syns per serving**
original **3½**
green **10½**

Fry Light for spraying
4 red onions, peeled and quartered
4 lean pork loin chops, all visible fat removed
2 garlic cloves, peeled and sliced
3 apples, cored and quartered
2 carrots, peeled and thickly sliced
4 celery stalks, thickly sliced
1 tbsp chopped sage leaves
salt and freshly ground black pepper

500ml/16fl oz chicken stock made from Bovril
2 level tbsp cornflour

for the mash:
800g/1lb 12oz swede, peeled and roughly chopped
200g/7oz very low fat natural fromage frais
2 tbsp chopped flat-leaf parsley
salt and freshly ground black pepper

Preheat the oven to 200°C/Gas 6. Spray an ovenproof casserole dish with Fry Light.

Place the onion quarters in the casserole dish with the pork chops, garlic, apples, carrots, celery and sage. Season well.

Place the stock in a small saucepan and bring to the boil. Mix the cornflour with 2 tablespoons water to form a paste and stir into the stock. Remove from the heat. Pour over the meat, fruit and vegetable mixture, cover tightly and cook in the oven for 45–50 minutes or until the meat is tender.

Meanwhile, make the mash by boiling the swede in a large pan of boiling, lightly salted water until tender. Drain, return to the pan and mash until fairly smooth. Stir in the fromage frais and parsley and season well. To serve, divide the casserole between four warmed plates and serve with the swede mash.

**BONUS POINT**
You can substitute celeriac for the swede if desired.

119

serves 4
**preparation time**
10 minutes
**cooking time**
15–20 minutes
**syns per serving**
original **free**
green **10**

# Pork and mushroom stroganoff

Tender strips of pork are cooked gently with onions, garlic and mushrooms in this Free version of a classic dish.

**700g/1lb 10oz lean pork tenderloin**
  **(all visible fat removed)**
**Fry Light for spraying**
**8 small onions, peeled and halved**
**2 garlic cloves, peeled and crushed**
**200g/7oz button mushrooms, halved**
**200g/7oz large flat field or Portobello**
  **mushrooms, finely chopped**
**a pinch of grated nutmeg**
**400g/14oz very low fat natural**
  **yogurt**
**2 tbsp chopped gherkins**
**salt and freshly ground black pepper**

**to garnish:**
**chopped parsley**

■  Place the pork between two sheets of cling film and flatten with a mallet or rolling pin. Cut into thin strips and set aside.

■  Spray a non-stick frying pan with Fry Light and when hot add the onions and garlic and stir-fry for 3–4 minutes. Add the mushrooms and stir-fry over a high heat for 3–4 minutes. Then add the nutmeg and the pork and cook over a high heat for 5–7 minutes until cooked through.

■  Whisk the yogurt until smooth and stir into the pork mixture with the gherkins and heat through without boiling. Season and sprinkle over chopped parsley to garnish. Serve immediately.

**BONUS POINT**
For variety, use chicken or beef in this recipe instead of the pork.

# Luxury chilli con carne

The ultimate food for in front of the telly. This dish tastes even better the next day when the flavours have melded.

serves 4
preparation time
15 minutes
cooking time
about 1 hour 10
minutes
syns per serving
original 5½
green 16½

Fry Light for spraying
1 onion, peeled and finely chopped
3 garlic cloves, peeled and crushed
1 tsp dried chilli flakes
3 tsp ground cumin
1 tsp ground coriander
1 tsp sweet smoked paprika
700g/1lb 10oz extra lean minced beef
300g/10oz button mushrooms, halved
2 x 400g/14oz cans chopped tomatoes
2–3 tbsp artificial sweetener
2 level tbsp tomato purée

bay leaf
salt and freshly ground black pepper
1 x 400g/14oz can red kidney beans, drained and rinsed

to serve:
chopped coriander leaves
finely sliced spring onion
finely diced red pepper
very low fat natural fromage frais
finely diced cucumber
wedges of lime
boiled white rice (optional)

Preheat the oven to 200°C/Gas 6. Spray a flame- and ovenproof casserole dish with Fry Light. Place over a high heat and add the onions. Stir-fry for 3–4 minutes and then add the garlic, chilli flakes, cumin, coriander, paprika and beef. Stir-fry for 4–5 minutes and then add the mushrooms, tomatoes, sweetener, tomato purée and bay leaf.

Bring to the boil, season well, cover tightly and place in the oven to cook for 1 hour. Remove from the oven and stir in the kidney beans. Place on top of the hob and cook gently for 8–10 minutes, stirring occasionally.

To serve, ladle the chilli into warmed serving bowls and sprinkle each serving with the coriander, spring onions and red pepper together with a dollop of fromage frais, finely diced cucumber and lime wedges. Serve with boiled white rice, if desired (on an Original day, this counts as 2 Syns per 30g/1oz cooked weight).

**BONUS POINT**
Serve spoonfuls of the chilli on crisp lettuce leaves as a starter or quick snack.

ORIGINAL

**serves** 4
**preparation time**
15 minutes + 3–4
hours marinating
**cooking time**
30 minutes
**syns per serving**
original **free**
green **6**

# Lemon and rosemary lamb skewers with aubergine purée

In the summer, try cooking these delicious skewers over a barbecue for an extra special flavour.

**350g/12oz lean lamb fillet, cut into
  bite-sized pieces**

**for the marinade:**
**3 garlic cloves, peeled and crushed**
**2 tbsp chopped rosemary leaves**
**juice of 1 lemon**
**100g/3½oz very low fat natural
  yogurt**
**2 tsp finely grated lemon zest**
**salt and freshly ground black pepper**

**for the purée:**
**2 large aubergines**
**1 garlic clove, peeled and crushed**

**6 spring onions, finely chopped**
**juice of 1 lemon**
**8–9 tbsp finely chopped mint leaves**
**6 plum tomatoes, deseeded and
  finely chopped**
**2 red peppers, deseeded and cut into
  bite-sized pieces**

**to serve:**
**crisp green lettuce leaves**
**sliced red onion**
**sliced cucumber**

■ Put the lamb in a mixing bowl. Mix together the marinade ingredients, add to the lamb, season and toss. Cover and leave to marinate for a few hours in the fridge. Preheat the oven to 220°C/Gas 7. Prick the aubergine skins all over with a fork, place on a non-stick baking sheet and bake for 25–30 minutes or until the aubergines are soft. Remove and cover with foil until cool enough to handle.

■ Halve the aubergines and scoop the flesh into a food processor. Add the garlic, spring onions, lemon juice and mint leaves. Season and blend until fairly smooth. Transfer to a bowl and stir in the tomatoes. Set aside. Preheat the grill to hot. Thread the lamb and red pepper onto eight skewers and grill for 7–8 minutes, turning once, until lightly browned. To serve, place two skewers on each plate with a portion of the purée and accompany with lettuce leaves, sliced red onion and cucumber.

**BONUS POINT**
If you are using
bamboo skewers,
soak them in
water before
threading the food
onto them.

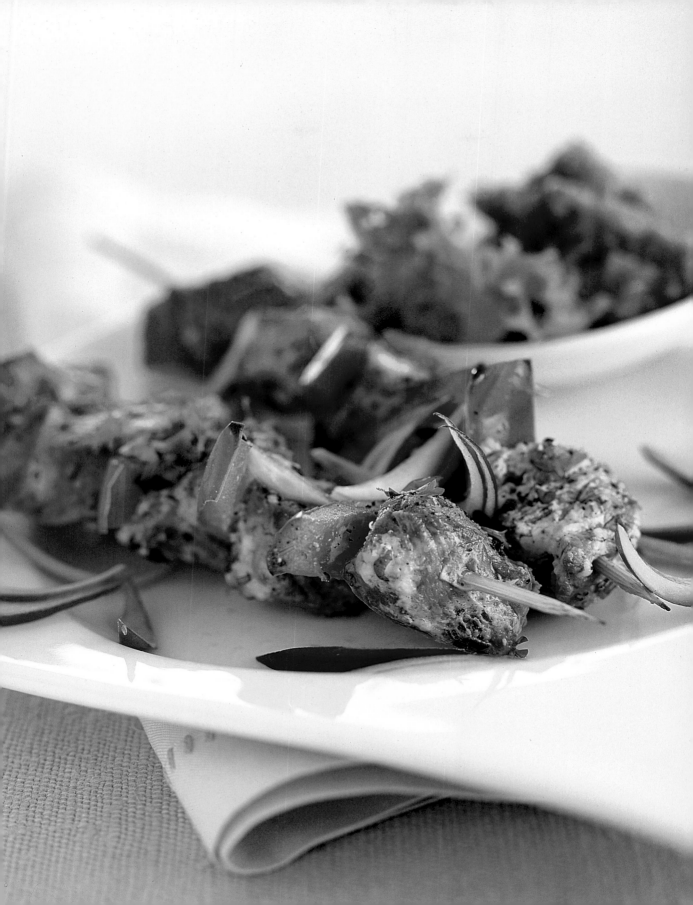

# Oriental beef and mixed pepper stir-fry

serves 4
**preparation time**
20 minutes
**cooking time**
about 15 minutes
**syns per serving**
original **free**
green **9**

The sweet juicy flavours of the peppers marry well with the strips of beef and oriental sauces in this quick-to-prepare family supper.

Fry Light for spraying

500g/1lb 2oz beef sirloin steak (all visible fat removed), cut into thin strips

6 spring onions, cut into 6cm/2¼in lengths

2 garlic cloves, peeled and finely sliced

1 red chilli, deseeded and finely sliced or chopped

3 tsp finely chopped lemongrass

2.5cm/1in piece of ginger, peeled and cut into thin slivers

1 yellow pepper, deseeded and very thinly sliced

1 orange pepper, deseeded and very thinly sliced

1 red pepper, deseeded and very thinly sliced

60g/2oz bean sprouts

2 tbsp red wine vinegar

2 tbsp dark soy sauce

1 tbsp fish sauce

1 tbsp sweet chilli sauce

4–5 tbsp chopped coriander leaves

juice of 2 limes

■ Spray a large, non-stick wok or frying pan with Fry Light. Place over a high heat and add the beef strips. Stir-fry for 4–5 minutes until the meat is browned and tender and then remove from the pan, set aside and keep warm. Wipe out the pan with kitchen paper and re-spray with Fry Light.

■ Heat the pan and add the spring onions, garlic, chilli, lemongrass and ginger to the pan and stir-fry for 1–2 minutes, before adding the peppers and the bean sprouts. Stir-fry for 3–4 minutes and then add the vinegar, soy, fish and sweet chilli sauces, 90ml/3fl oz water and the beef. Stir and continue to fry for 2–3 minutes.

■ Remove from the heat and stir in the coriander leaves and lime juice. Pile into four warmed serving bowls and serve immediately.

**BONUS POINT**
If your steak is very thick, place between two sheets of cling film and use a mallet or rolling pin to beat the steak until it is about 1.5cm/¾in thick.

# Italian-style spaghetti and meatballs

This delicious dish of meatballs spiked with garlic, ginger and herbs and tossed in an aromatic tomato sauce is perfect for a replenishing supper.

**serves** 4
**preparation time**
15 minutes
+ 2–3 hours
chilling
**cooking time**
about 40 minutes
**syns per serving**
original **15**
green **11½**

for the meatballs:
2 tsp garlic salt
2 tsp ground ginger
500g/1lb 2oz extra lean minced beef
4 spring onions, very finely chopped
1 small egg, lightly beaten
2 tbsp mixed chopped herbs (parsley, oregano and basil)
salt and freshly ground black pepper

2 onions, peeled and finely chopped
1 x 400g/14oz can chopped tomatoes
1 courgette, finely diced
2 garlic cloves, peeled and crushed

2 tbsp chopped basil
1–2 tbsp artificial sweetener
250ml/8fl oz beef stock made from Bovril
salt and freshly ground black pepper
350g/12oz dried wholemeal spaghetti

to garnish:
basil leaves

GREEN

■ Make the meatballs by combining all the ingredients in a mixing bowl and then, using your fingers, mix thoroughly to combine. Cover and chill for 2–3 hours or overnight to let the flavours develop.

■ Place the onions in a large saucepan with the tomatoes, courgette, garlic, basil, sweetener and stock. Bring to the boil, reduce the heat and simmer gently for 10–12 minutes. Season and keep hot.

■ Divide the meat mixture into 24 portions and shape each one into a ball. Add to the tomato mixture, cover and cook gently for 20–25 minutes, stirring occasionally, until the meat is cooked through and tender.

■ Cook the spaghetti according to the packet instructions. To serve, divide the spaghetti between four warmed shallow bowls or plates and top with the meatballs and sauce. Garnish with basil leaves and serve.

**BONUS POINT**
Try varying the flavour of this dish by using minced pork or chicken, or a mixture of both.

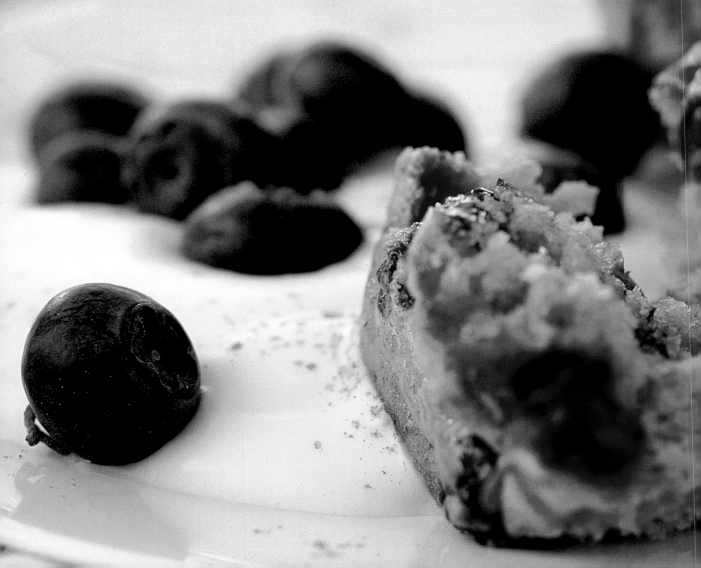

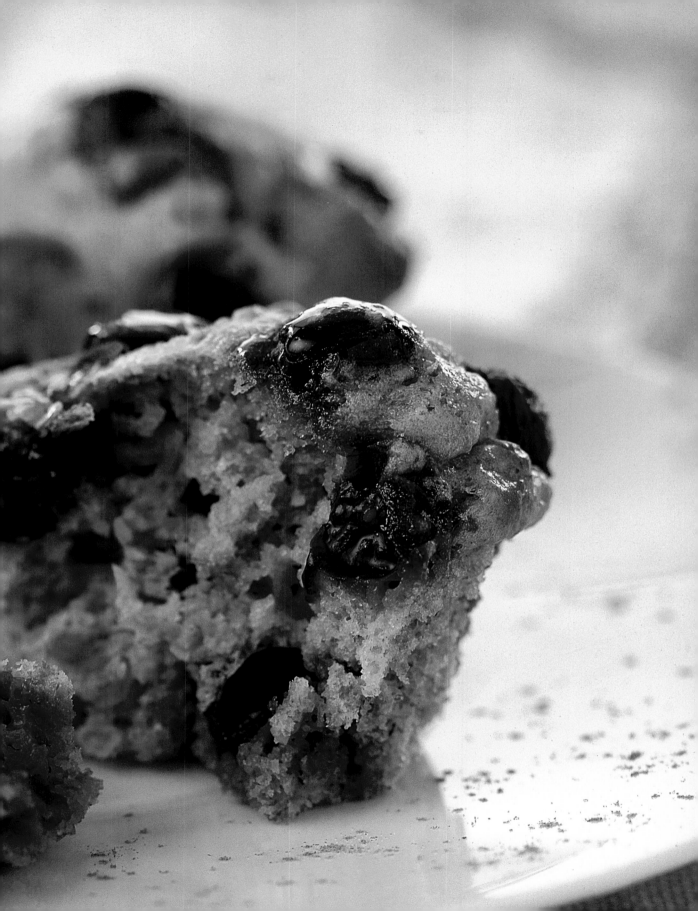

# Vegetable samosas with mint chutney

serves 4
(makes 12)
**preparation time**
20 minutes
**cooking time**
35–40 minutes
**syns per serving**
original **3**
green **3**

**GREEN/ORIGINAL**

**for the samosas:**
Fry Light for spraying
1 small onion, peeled and chopped
1 tsp finely grated garlic
1 tsp finely grated ginger
1 tsp ground cumin
1 tsp hot curry powder
200g/7oz mixed carrots, swede and
    courgette cut into 1cm/½in cubes
salt
juice of 1 lemon
3 tbsp chopped coriander leaves

6 small sheets of fresh filo pastry

**for the chutney:**
300g/10oz very low fat natural
    fromage frais
1 green chilli, deseeded and chopped
6 tbsp finely chopped coriander
leaves
3 tbsp finely chopped mint leaves
2–3 tbsp artificial sweetener
juice of 1 lime

■ Spray a large, non-stick frying pan with Fry Light and place over a medium heat. Add the onion, garlic and ginger and stir-fry for 3–4 minutes. Add the cumin and curry powder with the diced vegetables and 2–3 tablespoons of water and cook over a high heat, stirring often, for 4–5 minutes or until the vegetables are just tender. Season and stir in the lemon juice and coriander leaves. Set aside to cool.

■ Preheat the oven to 190°C/Gas 5. Line a baking sheet with non-stick baking parchment and lightly spray with Fry Light. Cut each filo sheet in half lengthways and place on a work surface. Lightly spray with Fry Light. Place a spoonful of the filling at one end of a filo strip and on one side only. Fold the empty corner of the pastry over the filling to make a triangle. Continue to enclose the filling by rolling the triangle along the length of the filo. Repeat with the remaining filling and filo strips to give you 12 samosas. Place on the baking sheet, spray with Fry Light and bake in the oven for 12–15 minutes until crisp and golden.

■ Meanwhile, make the chutney by placing all the ingredients in a food processor and blend until smooth. Season and chill until required. Serve the hot samosas with the chutney, garnished with coriander leaves.

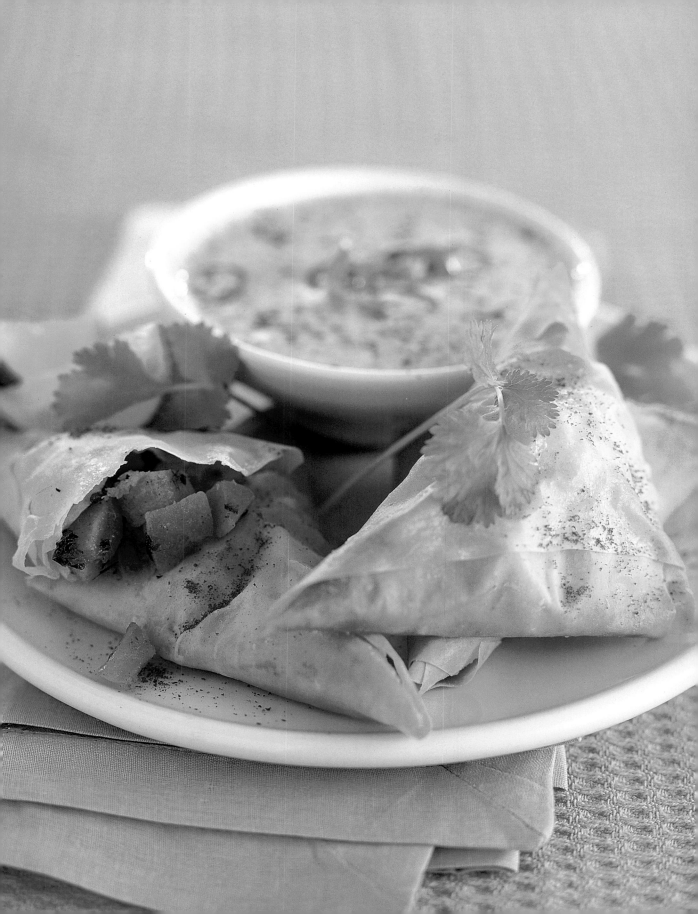

**serves** 4
**preparation time**
15 minutes
**cooking time**
1 hour
**vegetarian**
**syns per serving**
original **8**
green **free**

GREEN

# Crispy stuffed potato skins

These scooped-out jacket potatoes are filled with a fresh, colourful and crunchy mix of vegetables and herbs.

4 x 225g/8oz baking potatoes
Fry Light for spraying
sea salt

for the stuffing:
4 spring onions, finely sliced
3 plum tomatoes, deseeded and
   finely chopped
4 tbsp chopped coriander leaves

1 red chilli, deseeded and finely
   chopped
juice of 1 lime
salt and freshly ground black pepper

to serve:
very low fat natural yogurt (optional)
chopped coriander leaves

■ Preheat the oven to 200°C/Gas 6. Scrub the potatoes and place on a baking sheet. Lightly spray each one with Fry Light and bake for 1 hour or until tender.

■ Meanwhile, make the stuffing by mixing the spring onions, tomatoes, coriander and chilli in a bowl. Add the lime juice and season well. Set the stuffing to one side.

■ Using a sharp knife, cut each potato into four wedges and using a teaspoon, scoop out most of the flesh, leaving a thin layer of potato around the inside of each shell. Set the scooped-out potato to one side. Season the insides of each shell with sea salt and place on a serving plate or tray.

■ To serve, spoon the stuffing between the potato shells and top with a dollop of the yogurt, if desired. Garnish with chopped coriander leaves.

**BONUS POINT**
Use the scooped-out potato for a nice creamy mash or the topping for a vegetable pie.

# Toasted **triple** decker

Contrasting fillings – creamy egg and crunchy fresh vegetables – give these sandwiches an unusual twist.

**serves** 4
**preparation time**
15 minutes
**cooking time**
6–8 minutes
**vegetarian**
**syns per serving**
original **3**
green **3**

4 large eggs
200g/7oz very low fat natural
    fromage frais
1 tsp mustard powder
2 spring onions, finely sliced
2 tbsp chopped chives
salt and freshly ground black pepper
6 slices of wholemeal Nimble bread
3 ripe tomatoes, thinly sliced

1 large carrot, coarsely grated
a large handful of baby spinach
    leaves

■ Place the eggs in a pan of water and bring to the boil. Boil for 5–6 minutes and then plunge into cold water. Carefully peel the shells, place in a bowl and roughly mash with a fork. In a separate bowl, mix together the fromage frais and mustard powder and add to the eggs with the spring onions and chives. Season and set aside.

■ Lightly toast the slices of bread. Place one slice of toast on a board and top with half the tomato slices, carrots and spinach leaves. Add a second slice of toast on top of the vegetables and spread half the egg mixture over it. Finish by topping with a third slice and press down gently. Using a sharp bread knife, cut the sandwich diagonally into two. Repeat with the remaining three slices and fillings. If taking on a picnic or using for a lunch box, wrap tightly in cling film.

**BONUS POINT**
Use a variety of
vegetable fillings
to ring a change to
these sandwiches.

GREEN/ORIGINAL

serves 4
**preparation time**
20 minutes
**cooking time**
about 45 minutes
**vegetarian**
**syns per serving**
original **6**
green **3¹⁄₂**

GREEN

# Tex-mex chilli burritos

Pure comfort food, this warming and filling dish will be a favourite tea-time treat for the whole family.

Fry Light for spraying
1 red onion, peeled and chopped
2 garlic cloves, peeled and
   crushed
1 tsp ground cumin
1 red pepper, deseeded and very
   finely diced
1 red chilli, deseeded and finely
   sliced
1 x 400g/14oz can chopped tomatoes

1 x 200g/7oz can red kidney beans,
   drained
2–3 tbsp artificial sweetener
salt and freshly ground black pepper
4 x 30g/1oz soft flour tortillas
5 tbsp very low fat natural yogurt

to garnish:
chopped coriander leaves

■ Spray a large, non-stick frying pan with Fry Light. Place over a medium heat and add the onions and garlic. Stir-fry for 3–4 minutes and then add the cumin, red pepper, red chilli and tomatoes. Bring to the boil and cook over a medium heat for 20 minutes or until thickened. Add the kidney beans and sweetener and cook for another 5 minutes. Season well.

■ Preheat the oven to 200°C/Gas 6 and lightly spray a small, shallow, ovenproof dish with Fry Light. Lay the tortillas on a clean work surface and spoon a couple of spoonfuls of the bean mixture into the centre of each one (keep a little leftover to use for the topping). Fold each tortilla to form a neat parcel, secure with a cocktail stick and place, seam side down, in the dish, to fit snugly. Spoon over the yogurt and top with the remaining bean and tomato mixture.

■ Place in the oven and bake for 10–12 minutes until lightly browned. Serve immediately, garnished with chopped coriander leaves. Remember to remove the cocktail sticks before serving.

**BONUS POINT**
You can make the chilli mixture a couple of days in advance and you will find the flavours improve on standing. Or freeze it and use within a month.

# Pea and tomato tortilla

Wonderful served warm or at room temperature, this tortilla makes a terrific tea-time snack, or serve for supper with a crisp green salad.

**serves** 4
**preparation time** 20 minutes
**cooking time** 30–45 minutes
**vegetarian**
**syns per serving** original **2** green **free**

**Fry Light for spraying**
**2 red onions, peeled and finely**
**    chopped**
**60ml/2fl oz vegetable stock**
**100g/3½ oz potatoes**
**6 plum tomatoes, deseeded**
**6 large eggs**
**salt and freshly ground black pepper**
**100g/3½ oz fresh or frozen peas**
**2 tbsp chopped flat-leaf parsley**

GREEN

■ Spray a medium-sized, non-stick frying pan with Fry Light. Place over a medium heat and add the onions and stock. Cook the onions gently for 5 minutes until the stock is absorbed and the onions are soft.

■ Meanwhile, peel and cut the potatoes into 1cm/½in cubes and deseed and cut the tomatoes into 1cm/½in pieces. Add to the onion mixture, turn the heat to high and stir-fry for 3–4 minutes.

■ Lightly beat the eggs, season well and pour into the frying pan along with the peas and parsley. Reduce the heat to low and cook gently for 12–15 minutes, or until the underside is browned and set.

■ Place the pan under a preheated hot grill and cook for 3–4 minutes until the top is set and golden brown. Remove and serve either warm or at room temperature, cut into wedges.

**BONUS POINT**
If you feel like a change, substitute chopped green beans for the peas.

# Sardinian-style vegetable pizza

serves 6
preparation time
about 50 minutes
cooking time
about 30 minutes
vegetarian
syns per serving
original 4
green 4

This crispy-based pizza, topped with tomatoes, courgettes, peppers and basil, will put a smile on the faces of children and grown-ups alike.

**for the base:**
1 x 145g sachet pizza base mix

**for the topping:**
1 x 400g/14oz can chopped tomatoes
3 tbsp chopped basil
4 garlic cloves, sliced
3 tbsp artificial sweetener

salt and freshly ground black pepper
1 courgette, thinly sliced
1 yellow pepper, deseeded and thinly sliced
1 red onion, peeled and thinly sliced

**to garnish:**
mixed chopped herbs

Prepare the pizza dough according to the packet instructions. Form into a ball and place in a bowl lightly sprayed with Fry Light, cover with a clean tea towel and let stand for 10–15 minutes.

Meanwhile, place the tomatoes, basil, garlic and sweetener in a saucepan and bring to the boil. Cover, reduce the heat and simmer gently for 25–30 minutes. Allow to cool and season. Preheat the oven to 200°C/Gas 6 and line a baking sheet with non-stick baking parchment.

Knead the dough and roll out into a large disc (about 30cm/12in in diameter) and place on the baking sheet. Spread the tomato sauce over the base, leaving a border around the edges, and arrange the courgette, pepper and onion on top. Season well and bake for 30 minutes. Serve immediately, garnished with chopped fresh herbs.

**BONUS POINT**
This pizza can be frozen once cooked and re-heated after being defrosted.

GREEN/ORIGINAL

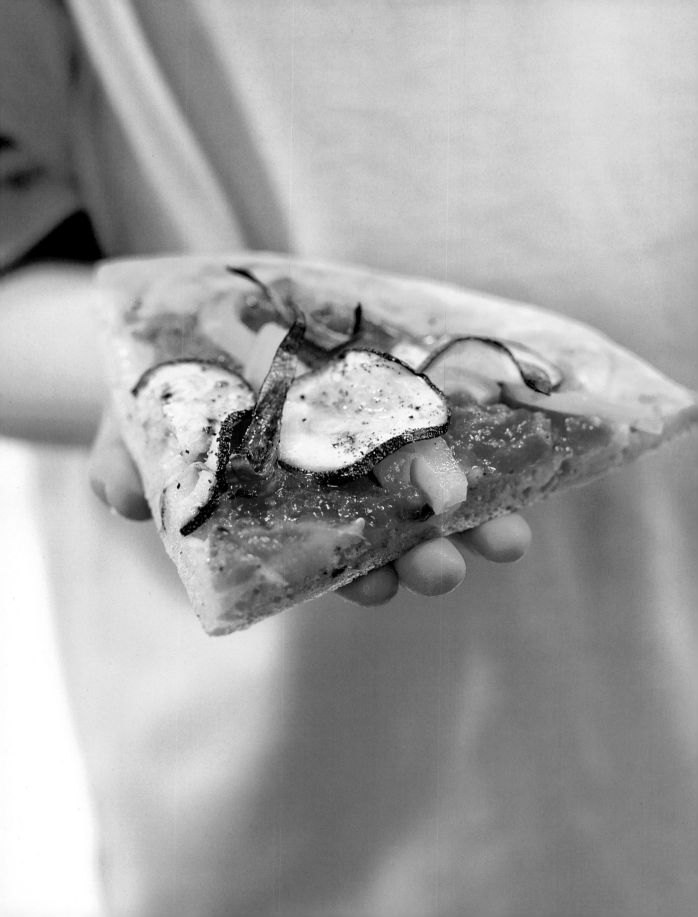

GREEN/ORIGINAL

**serves** 4
**preparation time**
15 minutes
**cooking time**
15 minutes
**vegetarian**
**syns per serving**
original **6½**
green **6½**

# Grilled pepper and olive bruschetta

A quick and tasty treat for tea-time, these colourful, Italian-style, vegetable-topped toasts will satisfy a rumbling tummy.

2 onions, peeled and thinly sliced
3 tbsp balsamic vinegar
100ml/3½fl oz vegetable stock
1 red pepper
1 yellow pepper
1 orange pepper

8 black olives, stoned and roughly chopped
4 x 60g/2oz slices wholemeal bread
2 garlic cloves, peeled and cut in half
salt and freshly ground black pepper

Place the onions, balsamic vinegar and stock in a large, non-stick frying pan and cook over a low heat for 6–8 minutes or until the liquid has been absorbed and the onions are browned.

Meanwhile, place the peppers under a hot grill and grill for 5–6 minutes, turning once until charred and blistered. Remove to a plastic bag for 10 minutes, then peel, deseed and roughly chop the flesh and place in a bowl with the onions and the olives.

Toast the slices of bread and place on a work surface. Rub each slice of bread with the halved garlic cloves. Mix together the pepper, onion and olive mixture. Season and divide among the four toasted slices of bread. Eat immediately.

**BONUS POINT**
If you do not have time to grill and peel the peppers, use the canned or bottled ones that are available in supermarkets.

# Irish potato cakes

These potato cakes are generously flavoured with spring onions, mustard and herbs. Serve with a crisp salad or steamed vegetables.

600g/1lb 6oz potatoes, peeled and
  roughly chopped
200g/7oz cabbage, very finely
  shredded
1 carrot, peeled and coarsely grated
4 spring onions, finely sliced

2 tbsp finely chopped dill
1 tbsp finely chopped parsley
1 level tsp wholegrain mustard
salt and freshly ground black pepper
Fry Light for spraying

serves 4
preparation time
30 minutes +
chillling
cooking time
about 16 minutes
vegetarian
syns per serving
original 5½
green free

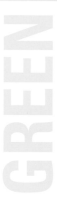

■ Place the potatoes in a pan of lightly salted boiling water and cook for 12–15 minutes or until tender. Drain and return to the pan. Mash until smooth and allow to cool.

■ Meanwhile, cook the cabbage and carrot in a pan of boiling water for 3–4 minutes, drain and add to the cooled potato mixture with the spring onions, dill, parsley and mustard. Season well, mix thoroughly, cover and chill for 3–4 hours in the fridge, or overnight if time permits.

■ To cook, spray a large, non-stick frying pan with Fry Light. Divide the potato mixture into eight portions and form each portion into a round, flat 'cake'. Place the frying pan over a medium heat and cook the cakes in batches for 3–4 minutes on each side or until lightly golden. Serve either hot or at room temperature with a crisp salad or steamed vegetables.

**BONUS POINT**
To be Free on an Original day, replace the potatoes with a celeriac mash.

**serves** 4
**preparation time**
20 minutes
+ 20 minutes
marinating time
**cooking time**
8–10 minutes
**syns per serving**
original **1**
green **8**

# Long Island seafood skewers with a basil and tomato dip

Served with a creamy dip, these juicy and succulent fish skewers are very low in Syns on an Original day.

500g/1lb 2oz thick white fish fillet
   (cod, halibut or rock fish), skinned
juice of 2 limes
2 garlic cloves, peeled and crushed
3 tbsp chopped dill
salt and freshly ground black pepper
4 spring onions
2 red peppers
1 yellow pepper

for the dip:
200g/7oz very low fat natural yogurt
1 level tbsp green pesto
1 plum tomato, finely chopped
5 tbsp finely chopped basil leaves
salt and freshly ground black pepper

to serve:
mixed salad leaves
lime wedges
dill sprigs (optional)

Cut the fish into bite-sized pieces and place in a mixing bowl. In a separate bowl, mix together the lime juice, garlic and dill and add to the fish. Add seasoning and toss to coat evenly. Cover and set aside for 15–20 minutes.

Meanwhile, cut the spring onions into 6cm/2¼in lengths. Deseed and cut the peppers into bite-sized pieces. Set aside.

Make the dip by mixing together all the ingredients in a bowl. Season and chill until ready to serve.

Preheat the grill to medium-high. Thread the fish, spring onion and peppers alternately onto eight metal or pre-soaked bamboo skewers. Cook the skewers under the grill for 8–10 minutes, turning occasionally, until the fish is cooked through and the vegetables are just tender and slightly charred. Serve the seafood skewers with mixed salad leaves and the basil and tomato dip. Garnish with lime wedges and dill, if desired.

**BONUS POINT**
These skewers are also terrific if accompanied by a fresh tomato salsa. Just finely chop 2 plum tomatoes and blitz in the blender with basil and spring onions and a little lemon juice.

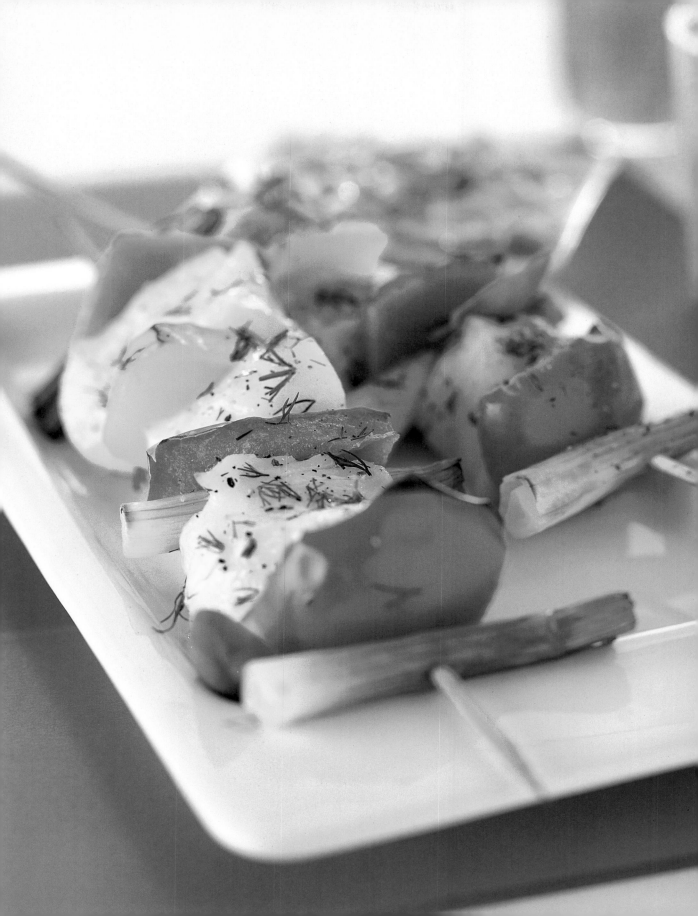

**serves** 4
**preparation time**
10 minutes +
4–5 hours
marinating
**cooking time**
20–25 minutes
**syns per serving**
original **2**
green **10**

ORIGINAL

# Spicy glazed chicken wings

Finger lickin' good, these sticky golden wings will leave you craving for more. They are perfect for cooking over a barbie in the summertime.

for the marinade:

4 tbsp light soy sauce

1 red chilli, finely chopped

3 tbsp clear honey

2 tsp English mustard powder

1 tsp finely grated ginger

1 tsp finely grated garlic

3 tbsp balsamic vinegar

2 level tbsp tomato purée

2 tsp cayenne pepper

16 large chicken wings, skinned

to serve:

salad leaves (optional)

◻ Place the light soy sauce, red chilli, honey, mustard powder, ginger, garlic, balsamic vinegar, tomato purée and cayenne pepper in a bowl and stir to mix well.

◻ Place the chicken wings in a wide, shallow mixing bowl. Pour over the marinade mixture and toss to coat well. Cover and marinate in the fridge for 4–5 hours, or overnight if time permits.

◻ Preheat the oven to 200°C/Gas 6. Line two baking sheets with non-stick baking parchment and place the chicken wings on them in a single layer. Brush them with any remaining marinade and then bake for 20–25 minutes until the chicken is cooked through and glazed. Serve with salad leaves, if desired.

**BONUS POINT**
Lean pork chops
are a good
substitute for the
chicken wings.
Use the same
marinade.

# Bangers and champ

Juicy sausages are cooked to perfection and served with this herby root vegetable mash – a most satisfying tea-time treat.

**serves** 4
**preparation time**
20 minutes
**cooking time**
30 minutes
**syns per serving**
original **5½**
green **9**

Fry Light for spraying
12 Bowyers 95% fat-free sausages
600g/1lb 4oz celeriac, peeled and cut
　　into small cubes
300g/10oz parsnips, peeled and cut
　　into small cubes
½ pointed or sweetheart cabbage,
　　cored and shredded
4 spring onions, finely sliced

6 tbsp very low fat natural yogurt
1 tsp English mustard powder
salt and freshly ground black pepper
3–4 tbsp chopped flat-leaf parsley

■ Preheat the oven to 200°C/Gas 6. Line a baking sheet with non-stick baking parchment and lightly spray with Fry Light. Place the sausages on it and bake for 20–25 minutes until cooked through and lightly browned.

■ Meanwhile, bring the celeriac and parsnips to the boil in a large saucepan of lightly salted water. Boil for 20–25 minutes or until very tender, drain and return to the saucepan. Cover with a lid and keep warm.

■ Spray a large, non-stick frying pan with Fry Light and when hot add the cabbage and spring onions. Stir-fry for 5–6 minutes and then add 75ml/2½fl oz water, cover and cook for 3–4 minutes until softened. Stir this mixture into the celeriac and parsnip mixture and roughly mash. Mix together the yogurt and mustard powder and add to the mash. Add seasoning and then the chopped parsley. Cover, set aside and keep warm.

■ To serve, divide the 'champ' between four warmed plates and top each serving with three sausages. Accompany with a selection of vegetables, if desired.

ORIGINAL

**BONUS POINT**
The champ can be made up to a day in advance; just heat thoroughly before serving.

GREEN/ORIGINAL

**serves** 6
**preparation time**
15 minutes
**cooking time**
15–20 minutes
**vegetarian**
**syns per muffin**
original **3**
green **3**

# Blueberry muffins

These delicious, sweet and tasty muffins are incredibly easy to prepare. You can readily substitute raspberries for the blueberries.

200g/7oz blueberries
30g/1oz All Bran, roughly crushed
2 tbsp artificial sweetener
60ml/2fl oz freshly squeezed orange
   juice
60g/2oz self-raising flour
2 level tsp baking powder

1 tsp ground cinnamon
$1/2$ tsp ground ginger
2 eggs, lightly beaten

to serve:
very low fat natural yogurt
blueberries (optional)

■ Preheat the oven to 200°C/Gas 6.

■ Place the blueberries, All Bran, sweetener and orange juice in a bowl and stir to mix well. Sift in the flour, baking powder and ground spices. Add the eggs and mix until fairly well blended.

■ Line six muffin tins with paper cases and spoon the mixture into them. Place in the oven and bake for 15–20 minutes until risen and firm to the touch. Remove from the oven and serve warm with a dollop of yogurt and blueberries, if desired.

**BONUS POINT**
These muffins will keep fresh in an airtight container for up to two days.

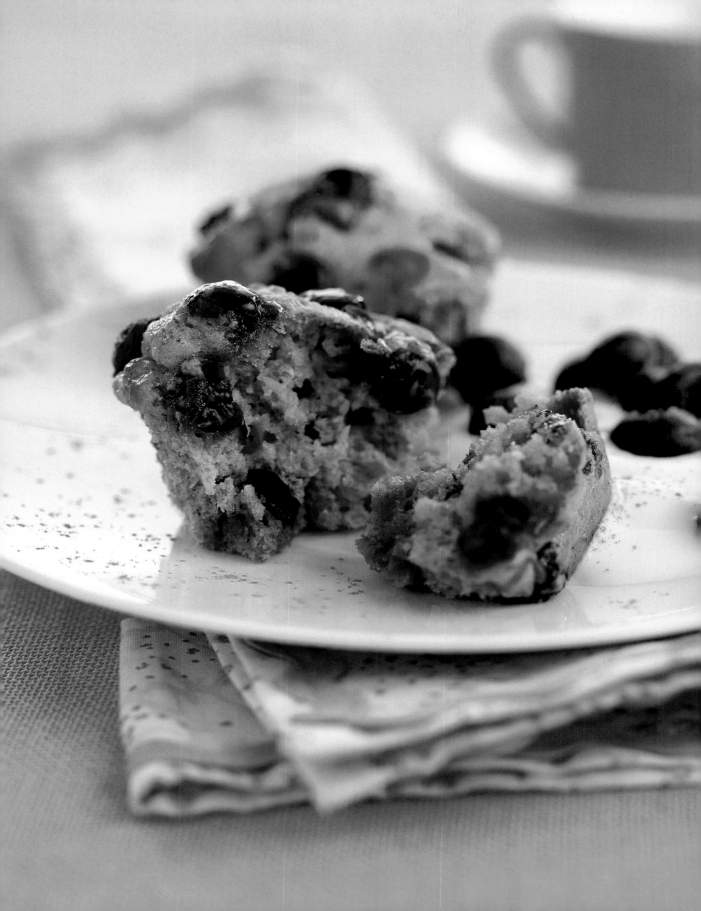

makes 12
scones
**preparation time**
20 minutes +
chilling
**cooking time**
10–12 minutes
**vegetarian**
**syns per scone**
original **3**
green **3**

## Strawberry and sultana scones

Eaten warm and straight from the oven, these scones are light and full of goodness. Serve them as a dessert with yogurt ice or ice cream.

**175g/6oz self-raising flour**
**¹/₂ level tsp baking powder**
**30g/1oz low fat spread**
**3–4 tbsp artificial sweetener**
**1 x 200g/7oz pot Müllerlight**
   **strawberry-flavoured yogurt**
**30g/1oz golden sultanas**

**Fry Light for spraying**

**to serve:**
**very low fat natural fromage frais**
**fresh strawberries**

■ Sift the flour into a mixing bowl with the baking powder. Add the low fat spread and sweetener and rub, using your fingers until the mixture resembles breadcrumbs. Add the yogurt and the sultanas and mix until the mixture forms a soft dough, adding a little extra flour if the dough is too sticky. Wrap in cling film and chill for 3–4 hours.

■ Preheat the oven to 220°C/Gas 7. Turn the dough out onto a lightly floured board and roll out to a 1.5cm/³/₄in thickness. Using a 4–5cm/2–2¹/₂in fluted biscuit cutter, cut into 12 rounds, re-rolling the excess pastry and using it up. Line a baking sheet with non-stick baking parchment and spray lightly with Fry Light. Using a palette knife, carefully place the pastry rounds on it and bake for 10–12 minutes or until risen and lightly browned. Serve immediately with the fromage frais and fresh strawberries.

**BONUS POINT**
Try using Müllerlight vanilla-flavoured yogurt to change the taste.

GREEN/ORIGINAL

# Mini citrus fruit bakewells

These tiny bite-sized delights are a great tea-time treat with their successful combination of flavours and contrasting textures.

**makes** 16
**preparation time**
15 minutes
**cooking time**
15–20 minutes
**vegetarian**
**syns per bakewell**
original **2½**
green **2½**

2 eggs
30g/1oz low fat spread
6 tbsp artificial sweetener
60g/2oz self-raising flour
3–4 drops almond extract
100g/3½ oz finely chopped mixed
   glacé citrus peel

for the topping:
4 level tsp icing sugar
a few drops of almond extract
a few drops of yellow food colouring

to garnish:
30g/1oz chopped mixed glacé citrus
   peel

Preheat the oven to 180°C/Gas 4 and line 16 mini muffin tins with paper cases.

In a mixing bowl, whisk together the eggs, low fat spread and artificial sweetener. Sieve in the flour and fold into the mixture with the almond extract and chopped peel.

Spoon into the paper cases to fill and bake for 15–20 minutes until firm and golden. Remove from the oven and cool.

While the bakewells are cooking, make the topping by mixing together the icing sugar, almond extract, yellow food colouring and a few drops of water in a small bowl until smooth. Drizzle the almond icing over each mini bakewell and top with chopped mixed peel.

**BONUS POINT**
Instead of the mixed peel, you can use chopped glacé cherries.

GREEN/ORIGINAL

**serves** 6
**preparation time**
15 minutes
**cooking time**
35-40 minutes
**vegetarian**
**syns per serving**
original **4¹/₂**
green **4¹/₂**

# Moist banana bread

This dreamy moist banana loaf is best eaten warm. Serve with a scoop of vanilla ice cream for the kids as a special treat.

2 ripe bananas
60g/2oz All Bran, roughly crushed
4 tbsp artificial sweetener
60ml/2fl oz apple juice
60g/2oz self-raising flour
5–6 drops vanilla essence
2 level tsp baking powder

¹/₂ tsp ground allspice
3 eggs, lightly beaten
salt

to serve:
very low fat natural yogurt or
    fromage frais (optional)

■ Preheat the oven to 200°C/Gas 6. Line a small, non-stick loaf tin with non-stick baking parchment.

■ Using a fork, roughly mash the bananas and place in a mixing bowl. Add the All Bran, sweetener and apple juice. Stir to mix well and then sift in the flour. Add the vanilla essence, baking powder and allspice and then stir in the beaten eggs and season with a pinch of salt. Mix until smooth and well blended.

■ Pour this mixture into the prepared loaf tin and bake for 35–40 minutes or until firm to the touch and golden brown. Remove from the oven and let cool in the tin for 10 minutes.

**BONUS POINT**
The loaf can be kept fresh for up to three days in an air-tight container. Then cut it into thick slices and toast for a yummy snack.

■ Remove from the tin and peel off the baking parchment. Cut into slices and serve immediately, accompanied with a dollop of very low fat yogurt or fromage frais, if desired.

GREEN/ORIGINAL

# Gingerbread squares

Flavoured with ginger and other spices, these tea-time treats are really delicious on their own or served with fruit and very low fat yogurt.

makes about 30 squares
preparation time 15 minutes
cooking time 30–35 minutes
vegetarian
syns per square
original 3½
green 3½

Fry Light for spraying
350g/12oz self-raising flour
175g/6oz golden caster sugar
100g/3½ oz low fat spread
1 egg
1 x 200g/7oz pot Müllerlight vanilla-flavoured yogurt

4–5 drops vanilla essence
2 tsp ground cinnamon
3 tsp ground ginger
salt
2 level tbsp candied ginger, finely chopped

Preheat the oven to 190°C/Gas 5. Spray an 18 x 30cm/7 x 12in (approximately) non-stick baking tin with Fry Light and line with non-stick baking parchment.

Sift the flour into a food processor and then add the caster sugar, low fat spread, egg, yogurt, vanilla essence, cinnamon and ground ginger. Season with a pinch of salt and process until smooth.

Spoon the mixture into the baking tin and smooth the top with the back of a spoon. Sprinkle over the candied ginger and bake for 30–35 minutes or until lightly golden and firm to the touch.

Take out of the oven and allow to cool for 5–10 minutes and then remove carefully from the tin and peel off the baking paper. Place on a board and cut into approximately 30 squares. Serve warm or at room temperature.

**BONUS POINT**
For a dessert, cut the slab of gingerbread into thin slices or wedges and serve it with low fat custard or very low fat natural fromage frais.

147

**makes** about 20 cookies
**preparation time** 25 minutes + chilling
**cooking time** 10–12 minutes
**vegetarian**
**syns per cookie**
original **2½**
green **2½**

# White and dark chocolate chip cookies

For a spicier version of these more-ish cookies, add a large pinch of ground cinnamon and ground ginger to the mixture before cooking.

60g/2oz self-raising flour
110g/4oz plain flour
40g/1½ oz low fat spread
100g/3½ oz Müllerlight toffee-flavoured yogurt
3–4 tbsp artificial sweetener
3–4 drops vanilla essence
1 tsp finely grated orange zest

Fry Light for spraying
15g/½ oz white chocolate, cut into small pieces
15g/½ oz dark chocolate, cut into small pieces

Sift the flours into a large bowl and rub in the low fat spread until the mixture resembles breadcrumbs.

Add the yogurt, sweetener, vanilla essence and orange zest and knead until the mixture forms a soft dough (adding a little extra flour if necessary (1 Syn per 1 level tsp), if the dough is too sticky. Form into a ball, wrap in cling film and chill for 5–6 hours or overnight if time permits.

Preheat the oven to 220°C/Gas 7. Line two baking sheets with non-stick baking parchment and spray lightly with Fry Light.

Turn the dough out onto a lightly floured surface and roll out to a thickness of a pound coin. Using a 4cm/1½in biscuit cutter, cut out 20 rounds, re-rolling the excess dough and using it up. Using a palette knife, carefully place the cookie rounds on the baking sheets.

Sprinkle over the white and dark chocolate on the surface of each cookie and bake for 10–12 minutes or until the cookies have slightly risen and lightly browned. Carefully remove to a wire rack and serve when cool.

GREEN/ORIGINAL

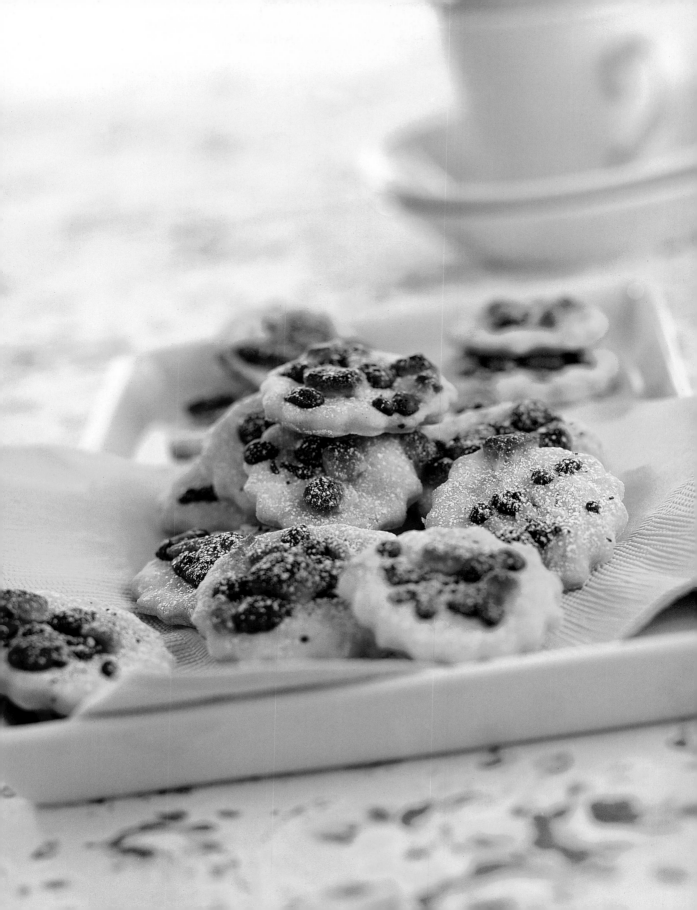

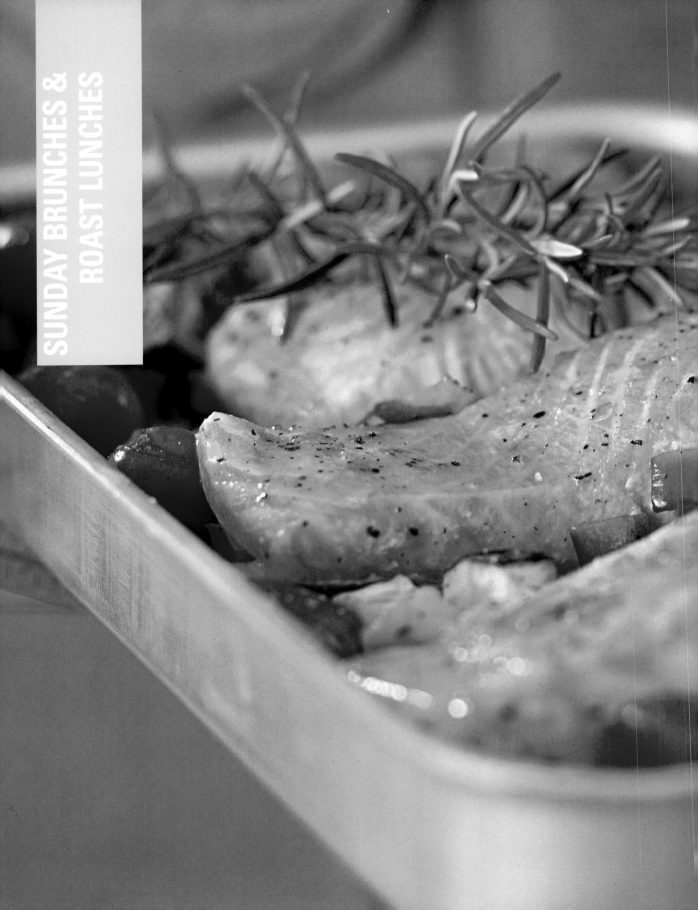

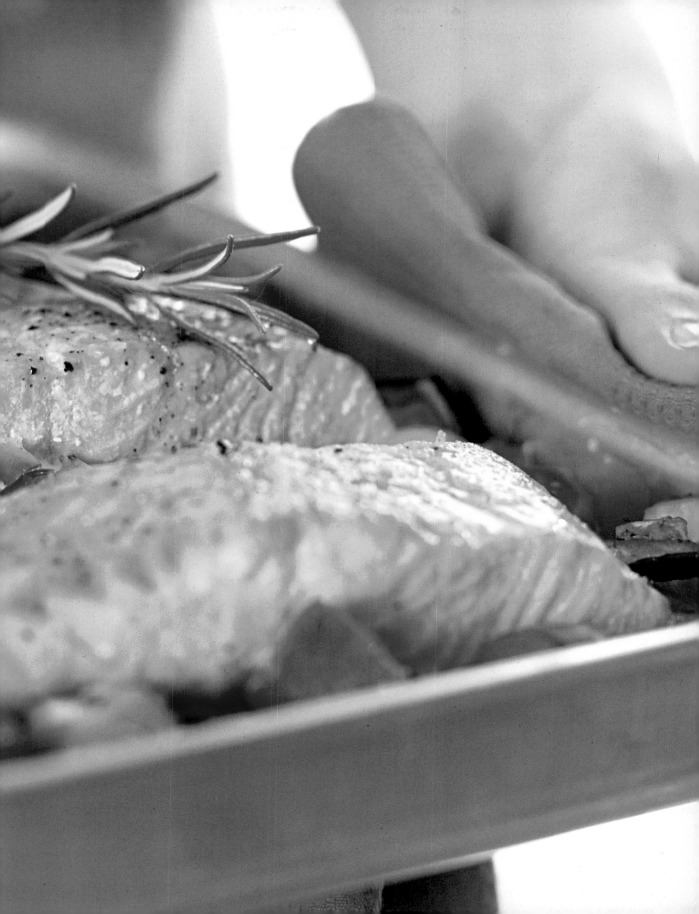

**serves** 4
**preparation time**
20 minutes
**syns per serving**
original **6½**
green **9½**

# Eggs benedict

A wonderful start to a lazy Sunday, this classic brunch dish of poached eggs over spinach and ham is served with a creamy herbed sauce.

for the sauce:
**10 tbsp very low fat natural
   fromage frais**
**60ml/2fl oz hot stock made from
   Bovril**
**1 tbsp very finely snipped chives**
**1 tbsp very finely chopped parsley**
**1 level tsp Dijon mustard**
**salt and freshly ground black pepper**

**1–2 tsp white wine vinegar**
**4 eggs**
**300g/10oz young leaf or baby
   spinach**

**1 tsp olive oil**
**juice of 1 lemon**
**4 x 60g/2oz slices of wholemeal
   toast**
**8 slices of ham (all visible fat
   removed)**

to serve:
**vine roasted plum tomatoes**

■   Make the sauce by combining all the ingredients in a food processor and blending until smooth. Season, set aside and keep warm.

■   Bring a large pan of lightly salted water to the boil. Stir in the vinegar, reduce the heat to a very gentle simmer and carefully break the eggs into the water. Cover the pan and let the eggs poach on a very low heat for about 4 minutes. Remove from the heat and carefully transfer the eggs to a large bowl of cold water.

**BONUS POINT**
Instead of the poached eggs, serve this dish with softly scrambled eggs for a change.

■   Meanwhile, place the spinach, olive oil and lemon juice in a non-stick pan and heat gently until the spinach is just wilted. Season to taste. To serve, place a slice of wholemeal toast on a warmed serving plate and top with the ham and spinach. Top each with a poached egg and spoon over the sauce. Serve immediately with vine roasted plum tomatoes.

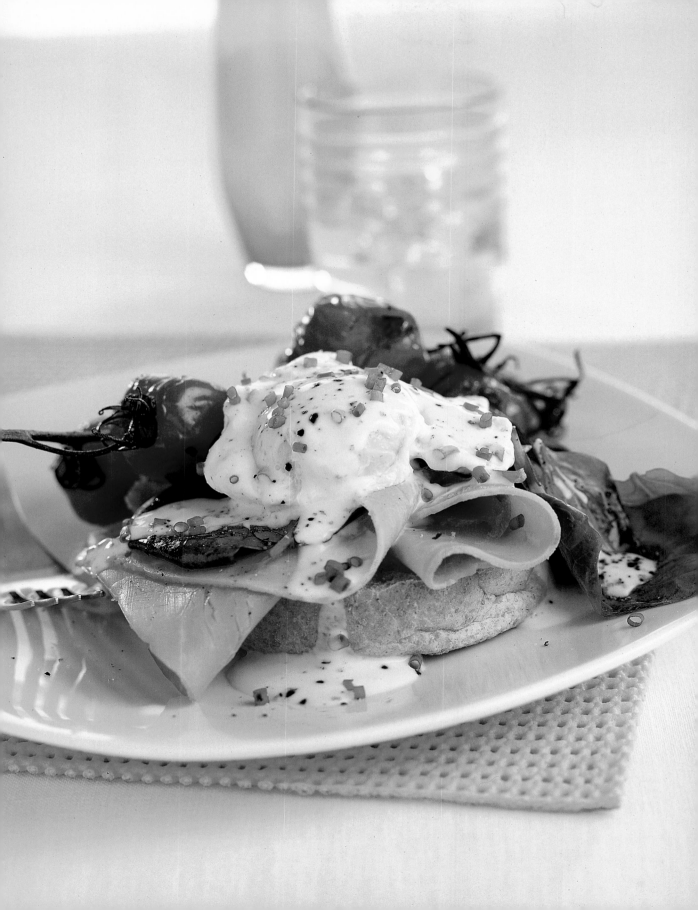

**serves** 4
**preparation time**
15 minutes
**cooking time**
25–30 minutes
**vegetarian**
**syns per serving**
original **6**
green **free**

GREEN

# Sweet potato wedges with chilli 'mayo'

Hot, sweet and spicy, these delicious wedges of sweet potato are perfectly complemented with a cool, creamy dip.

4 sweet potatoes (approximately 175g/6oz each)
1 tbsp coriander seeds
1 tbsp cumin seeds
1 tsp nigella seeds
1/2 tsp dried red chilli flakes
4 tbsp very low fat natural yogurt
juice of 1 lemon
sea salt
Fry Light for spraying

for the 'mayo':
200g/7oz very low fat natural fromage frais
1 tbsp sweet chilli sauce
1 tbsp light soy sauce
2 tbsp finely chopped coriander leaves
1 red chilli, deseeded and finely chopped

■ Preheat the oven to 200°C/Gas 6.

■ Peel the sweet potatoes and cut lengthways into 4–5 chunky wedges. Place in a shallow bowl. Lightly crush the coriander and cumin seeds in a mortar and pestle and place in a small bowl with the nigella seeds, dried chilli flakes, yogurt and lemon juice. Season and pour this mixture over the sweet potato wedges and toss to coat evenly.

■ Line a baking sheet with non-stick baking parchment and lightly spray with Fry Light. Arrange the potato wedges in a single layer and spray lightly with Fry Light. Place in the oven and roast for 25–30 minutes or until just tender.

■ Meanwhile, make the 'mayo' by mixing all the ingredients in a small bowl. Chill until ready to serve.

■ Remove the wedges from the oven and place on a large platter and serve immediately with the bowl of chilli mayo to accompany.

**BONUS POINT**
If you don't have a mortar and pestle, crush the seeds by using a rolling pin on a chopping board.

# Apple, ginger and cinnamon milkshake

serves 4
preparation time
5 minutes
vegetarian
syns per serving
original 3$^1$/$_2$
green 3$^1$/$_2$

Wake up and smell the goodness of this milkshake with its unusual combination of flavours, which will definitely kick-start your Sunday.

800ml/1$^1$/$_4$pt skimmed milk
1 x 200g/7oz pot Müllerlight vanilla-
   flavoured yogurt
5 tbsp sugar-free apple squash
$^1$/$_4$ tsp ground ginger
$^1$/$_4$ tsp ground cinnamon
3 tbsp artificial sweetener

to serve:
crushed ice
apple slices
mint leaves

Place the milk, yogurt and apple squash into a blender. Add the ground ginger, ground cinnamon and the sweetener and blend until the mixture is frothy.

Fill four tall glasses with crushed ice and pour over the milkshake. Garnish with apple slices and mint leaves and serve immediately.

**BONUS POINT**
For a really thick shake, use very low fat natural yogurt instead of the milk.

GREEN/ORIGINAL

155

**serves** 4
**preparation time**
10 minutes
**cooking time**
20–30 minutes
**vegetarian**
**syns per serving**
original **7**
green **7**

# Pancake and fruit stack

These layered fruit and pancake stacks are not only very pretty to look at but really delicious to tuck into.

1 x 128g/4½ oz pack pancake batter mix
4 tbsp artificial sweetener
½ level tsp bicarbonate of soda
2 level tsp baking powder
a few drops of vanilla essence
1 tsp finely grated orange zest
2 large eggs

Fry Light for spraying
1 x 200g/7oz pot Müllerlight vanilla-flavoured yogurt

to serve:
400g/14oz mixed summer berries
2 tbsp maple syrup or clear honey

■ Place the batter mix in a large mixing bowl with the sweetener, bicarbonate of soda, baking powder, vanilla essence and orange zest. Lightly beat the eggs and add to the bowl and stir with a wooden spoon until well combined.

■ Spray a large, non-stick frying pan with Fry Light and place over a medium heat. Place two or three large spoonfuls of the batter onto the hot pan (making sure they do not touch each other). Cook the pancakes for 1–2 minutes on each side until puffed up and lightly golden. Remove and place them between greaseproof paper and keep warm while you make the rest. You should make eight pancakes in total.

■ To serve, place a pancake on a warmed serving plate and dollop over a spoonful of the yogurt. Spoon over the berry mixture and top with another pancake.

■ Repeat with the remaining pancakes, yogurt and berries to give you three more servings. Top with any remaining berries and drizzle over some maple syrup or clear honey and serve immediately.

GREEN/ORIGINAL

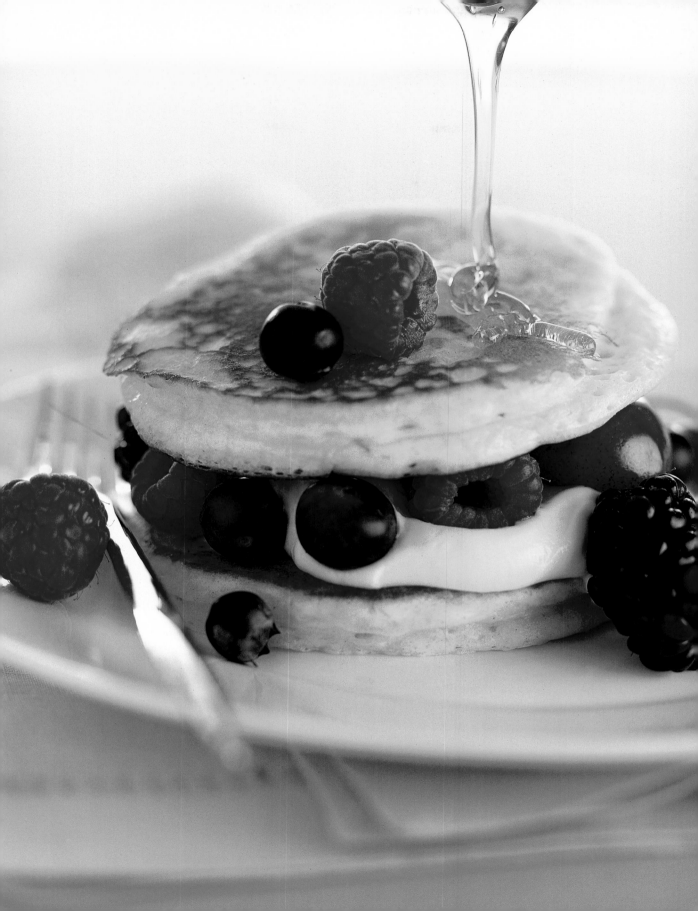

GREEN

serves 4
**preparation time**
15 minutes
**cooking time**
about 40 minutes
**vegetarian**
**syns per serving**
original **7**
green **free**

# Chunky root vegetable hot pot

A hearty one-pot dish of meltingly tender root vegetables cooked in a tomato-based stock, just perfect for a relaxed Sunday family lunch.

1 red onion, peeled and roughly
   chopped
4 stalks of celery, roughly sliced
450ml/¾pt vegetable stock
2 garlic cloves, peeled and thinly
   sliced
3 turnips, peeled and roughly
   chopped
2 carrots, peeled and roughly
   chopped
2 parsnips, peeled and roughly
   chopped

3 medium potatoes, peeled and cut
   into bite-sized pieces
60g/2oz red lentils
2 x 400g/14oz cans chopped
   tomatoes
300g/10oz small button mushrooms
2 sprigs of rosemary
salt and freshly ground black pepper

to garnish:
chopped parsley

■ Place the onion and celery and half the stock in a large saucepan. Bring to the boil, reduce the heat and simmer for 10 minutes.

■ Add the remaining stock with the garlic, turnips, carrots, parsnips and potatoes. Bring back to the boil and add the lentils, tomatoes, mushrooms and rosemary.

■ Bring the mixture back to the boil once again, reduce the heat, season well and simmer gently for 20–25 minutes or until the vegetables are tender. Sprinkle over some chopped parsley and serve immediately, ladled into warmed shallow bowls.

**BONUS POINT**
This dish can be frozen for up to a month.

# Cauliflower, chive and cheese gratin

A low-Syn version of cauliflower-cheese, this dish is perfect when entertaining as it is easy to prepare and is loved by family and friends.

**serves** 4
**preparation time**
15 minutes
**cooking time**
16–18 minutes
**vegetarian**
**syns per serving**
original **5**
green **5**

600g/1lb 6oz cauliflower
Fry Light for spraying
2 level tbsp cornflour
1 tsp dry English mustard
300ml/½pt skimmed milk
150g/5oz very low fat natural yogurt
60g/2oz reduced fat Cheddar cheese

4 tbsp finely chopped chives
salt and freshly ground black pepper

■ Wash the cauliflower and cut into florets. Bring a large saucepan of lightly salted water to the boil. Add the cauliflower florets to the pan and bring back to the boil. Reduce the heat and simmer gently for 5–6 minutes or until the florets are just tender. Drain and place in a medium-sized, shallow ovenproof dish that has been sprayed lightly with Fry Light. Set aside and keep warm.

■ Place the cornflour in a small bowl with the mustard powder and a couple of tablespoons of the milk. Mix until smooth. Grate the cheese.

■ Put the remaining milk in a small saucepan and bring to the boil. Stir in the cornflour and mustard mixture and cook gently for 2–3 minutes until thickened slightly. Remove from the heat and whisk in the yogurt and half the cheese. Stir in the chives and season well.

■ Preheat the grill to high. Pour the cheese and chive sauce over the cauliflower florets and sprinkle over the remaining cheese. Place under the grill for 5–6 minutes until lightly browned and bubbling. Serve immediately.

**BONUS POINT**
This dish can be frozen after it has been cooked. Defrost and heat thoroughly before serving.

GREEN/ORIGINAL

# Three kinds of mash

One recipe, three flavours: any of these mashes makes a really terrific accompaniment with grilled vegetables, meat or fish dishes.

## Creamy rocket and mustard mash

**serves** 4
**cooking time**
about 25 minutes
**vegetarian**
**syns per serving**
original 1/2
green 1/2

900g/2lb swede, peeled and cubed
200g/7oz very low fat natural
   fromage frais

2 level tsp wholegrain mustard
30g/1oz wild rocket, chopped
salt and freshly ground black pepper

■ Boil the swede in a large pan of lightly salted water for 12–15 minutes until tender. Drain and return to the pan. Add the fromage frais and mash until fairly smooth. Stir in the mustard and rocket, season well and serve.

## Spring onion, chive and butternut mash

**serves** 4
**cooking time**
about 20 minutes
**vegetarian**
**syns per serving**
original **free**
green **free**

900g/2lb butternut squash, peeled,
   deseeded and cut into small cubes
6 spring onions, very finely sliced

4 tbsp very finely snipped chives
salt and freshly ground black pepper

■ Boil the butternut squash in a large pan of lightly salted water for 15 minutes until tender. Drain and return to the pan. Mash until smooth and stir in the spring onions and chives to mix thoroughly. Season and serve.

## Chilli and coriander mash

**serves** 4
**cooking time**
about 20 minutes
**vegetarian**
**syns per serving**
original **8**
green **free**

900g/2lb potatoes, peeled and cut
   into small cubes
200g/7oz very low fat natural yogurt
1 tsp crushed garlic
1 red chilli, deseeded and finely
   chopped

6 tbsp chopped coriander leaves
1/2 tsp ground cumin
juice and finely grated zest of 1 lime
salt

■ Boil the potatoes in a large pan of lightly salted water for 12–15 minutes until tender. Drain and return to the pan. Add the yogurt and mash until smooth. Stir in the garlic, red chilli, coriander leaves, cumin and lime juice and zest. Mix well, season and serve.

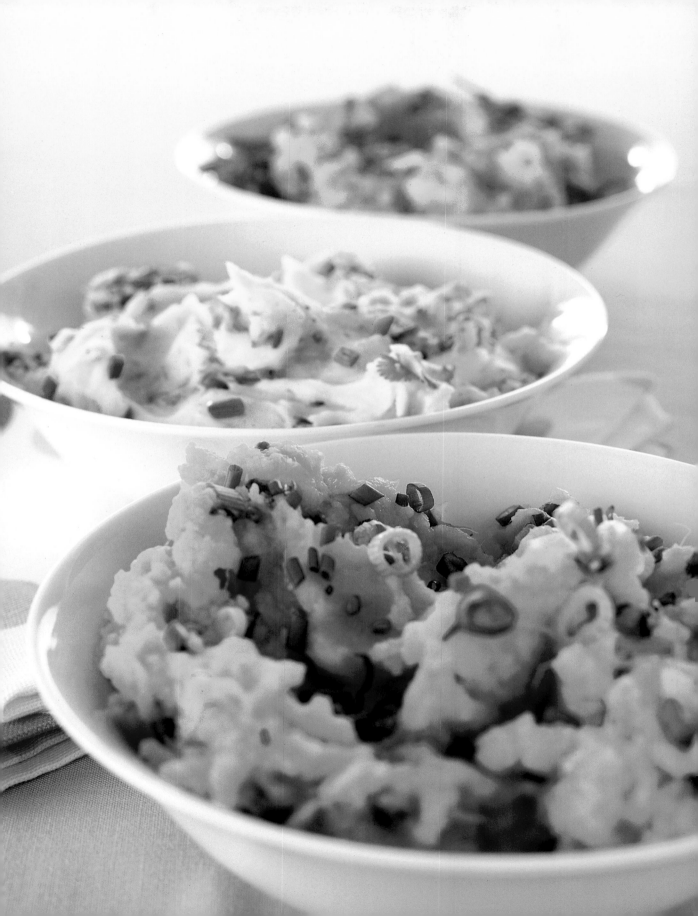

# Vegetable shepherd's pie

serves 4
**preparation time**
30 minutes
**cooking time**
25–30 minutes
**vegetarian**
**syns per serving**
original **9**
green **3½**

**GREEN**

Low in Syns on a Green day, this pie, cooked with Quorn and vegetables, makes a delicious, meat-free alternative to the traditional classic.

**for the topping:**
**600g/1lb 6oz potatoes (Desiree or**
   **King Edwards), peeled and cubed**
**400g/14oz celeriac, peeled and cubed**
**2 tbsp very low fat natural fromage**
   **frais**
**1 egg, beaten**
**100g/3½ oz reduced fat Cheddar**
   **cheese, grated**
**a pinch of grated nutmeg**
**salt and freshly ground black pepper**

**for the pie:**
**Fry Light for spraying**
**1 onion, peeled and finely chopped**
**2 garlic cloves, peeled and crushed**
**350g/12oz Quorn mince**
**1 x 400g/14oz can chopped tomatoes**
**500g/1lb 2oz frozen mixed**
   **vegetables, e.g. carrots, green**
**beans**
**3 tbsp soy sauce**
**Worcestershire sauce**
**freshly ground black pepper**

**to garnish:**

■ Make the topping for the pie by boiling the potatoes and celeriac in a large pan of lightly salted water for 15–20 minutes until tender. Drain, return to the saucepan and mash until fairly smooth. Stir in the fromage frais, egg, cheese and nutmeg. Season and set aside.

■ Preheat the oven to 180°C/Gas 4. Spray a large, non-stick saucepan with Fry light and cook the onions, garlic and Quorn mince for 5–6 minutes over a medium heat, stirring often. Add the tomatoes and cook for 20 minutes, stirring often. Stir in the vegetables and soy and Worcestershire sauces. Season with the black pepper. Pour into an ovenproof dish and spread the potato and celeriac mixture on top.

■ Place the dish in the oven and cook for 25–30 minutes until the topping is lightly browned. Serve immediately, garnished with chopped herbs.

**BONUS POINT**
This pie can easily be frozen; just heat thoroughly before serving.

# Spanish-style oven-baked vegetable rice

The flavours of Spain come together in this colourful rice dish, which can readily be prepared ahead of time. Heat thoroughly before serving.

**serves** 4
**preparation time**
20 minutes
**cooking time**
35–40 minutes
**vegetarian**
**syns per serving**
original **9½**
green **free**

175g/6oz easy-cook Basmati rice
a large pinch of saffron
Fry Light for spraying
2 red onions, peeled and finely chopped
3 garlic cloves, peeled and crushed
2 tsp sweet smoked paprika
4 baby leeks, thinly sliced
1 aubergine, roughly chopped
200g/7oz frozen or fresh peas
1 bay leaf
1 x 400g/14oz can chopped tomatoes
1 tbsp artificial sweetener

salt and freshly ground black pepper

to garnish:
chopped flat-leaf parsley

**GREEN**

■ Preheat the oven to 180°C/Gas 4. Cook the rice with the saffron in a large pan of lightly salted boiling water for 10–12 minutes or until just tender. Drain well and set aside.

■ Spray a large, non-stick frying pan with Fry Light and add the onions and garlic. Stir-fry over a medium heat for 2–3 minutes and then add the paprika, leeks and aubergine. Stir-fry for 2–3 minutes and then add the peas, bay leaf, chopped tomatoes and sweetener. Season well, cover and cook gently for 15–20 minutes or until the vegetables are just tender.

■ Remove the bay leaf from the vegetable mixture and then stir in the rice, mix well and transfer to a medium-sized ovenproof dish. Bake in the oven for 10 minutes. Serve immediately, garnished with chopped parsley, and accompany with a fresh cucumber salad.

**BONUS POINT**
This dish can be frozen or chilled in the fridge for 2–3 days in an air-tight container.

163

**serves** 4
**preparation time**
15 minutes
**cooking time**
15–20 minutes
**syns per serving**
original ½
green **15½**

# Honey and mustard roast salmon with roasted ratatouille

For a Sunday lunch treat, cook up this colourful and tasty roast fish dish. It is an impressive centrepiece to any table.

2 tsp finely grated lemon zest
juice of 2 lemons
1 tbsp clear honey
1 tsp mustard powder
salt and freshly ground black pepper
4 x 175g/6oz salmon fillets, skinned
Fry Light for spraying
250g/9oz cherry tomatoes
1 red pepper, deseeded and cut into
   1.5cm/¾in pieces
1 yellow pepper, deseeded and cut
   into 1.5cm/¾in pieces
1 small aubergine, cut into
   1.5cm/¾in pieces

2 small courgettes, cut into
   1.5cm/¾in pieces
2 red onions, peeled and cut into
   1.5cm/¾in pieces
3–4 garlic cloves, peeled and finely
   chopped
3 tbsp chopped rosemary
3 tbsp chopped basil
150ml/¼pt chicken stock made from
   Bovril

to garnish:
herb sprigs

ORIGINAL

▪ Preheat the oven to 200°C/Gas 6. Mix together the lemon zest and juice and the honey and mustard in a small bowl, season well and brush over the tops of the salmon fillets.

▪ Lightly spray a large, non-stick roasting tin with Fry Light. Place the vegetables in the tin, season and scatter over the garlic and herbs and then pour over the stock. Carefully place the salmon fillets on top of the vegetables. Cover with foil and bake for 15–20 minutes or until the salmon and vegetables are cooked through. Serve garnished with sprigs of rosemary or basil.

**BONUS POINT**
For added tang, sprinkle some balsamic vinegar over the vegetables before roasting them.

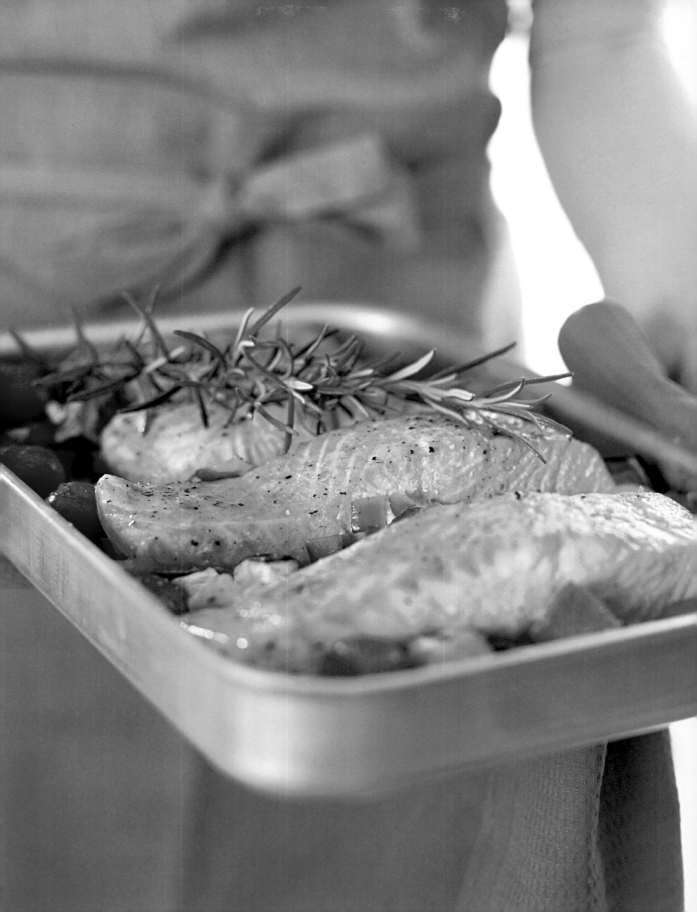

**serves** 4
**preparation time**
10 minutes +
4–5 hours
marinating
**cooking time**
20 minutes
**syns per serving**
original **free**
green 7$\frac{1}{2}$

# Roasted spiced pesto chicken

On a busy Sunday, this tasty chicken roast coated with a delicious pesto sauce takes no time at all to prepare.

**for the pesto:**
**10–12 tbsp chopped basil**
**4 tbsp balsamic vinegar**
**4 garlic cloves, peeled and crushed**
**60ml/2fl oz chicken stock made from Bovril**

**1 tsp dried red chilli flakes**
**salt and freshly ground black pepper**

**4 chicken breast fillets, skinned**
**Fry Light for spraying**

■ Make the pesto by placing the basil, balsamic vinegar, garlic, stock and chilli flakes in a food processor. Season and blend until fairly smooth.

■ Using a sharp knife, make 3–4 slashes on each chicken breast. Place the chicken in a shallow bowl in a single layer. Spoon over the pesto and rub the chicken well to coat. Cover and leave to marinate in the fridge for 4–5 hours, or overnight if time permits.

■ Preheat the oven to 190°C/Gas 5. Place the chicken breasts on a baking sheet, lightly sprayed with Fry Light. Roast the chicken in the oven for 20 minutes or until the chicken is cooked through and tender.

■ Slice each breast diagonally and serve accompanied by vegetables or a crisp radicchio salad.

**BONUS POINT**
Turkey steaks
would make a
good alternative
to the chicken.

# Citrus and garlic roasted poussins

An impressive addition to the Sunday roast lunch, these garlic, lemon and herb scented little poussins are packed with flavour.

**serves** 4
**preparation time**
20 minutes
**cooking time**
45–50 minutes
**syns per serving**
original **free**
green **10½**

4 small poussins (approximately 350–400g/12–14oz each)
4 large onions
6 tbsp finely chopped mixed herbs, e.g. tarragon, parsley, thyme
4 tbsp finely grated orange zest

4 tbsp finely grated lemon zest
6 garlic cloves, peeled and finely grated or crushed
juice of 1 lemon
salt and freshly ground black pepper
Fry Light for spraying

Preheat the oven to 200°C/Gas 6. Wash the poussins and dry them with kitchen paper. Peel the onions and cut each one into eight wedges and spread over the base of a large, non-stick baking tin. Place the poussins on top.

In a small bowl, mix together the herbs, orange and lemon zest, garlic and lemon juice. Spoon this mixture over the poussins to coat well. Season well, spray with Fry Light and place in the oven. Roast for 45–50 minutes or until the poussins are cooked through (the juices will run clear when a skewer is inserted into the thickest part of the thigh).

Remove from the oven, cover with foil and let the poussins rest for 10–12 minutes before serving. Remove the skin before eating and serve with the roasted onions and any green vegetables.

ORIGINAL

**BONUS POINT**
You could use two smallish chickens instead. Just remember to remove the skin before eating to keep your Syn count to a minimum.

**serves** 4
**preparation time**
15 minutes
**cooking time**
2 hours
**syns per serving**
original **2**
green **13**$^{1}/_{2}$

ORIGINAL

# Mediterranean lamb and carrot stew

A Middle Eastern-style lamb and vegetable stew, this rich and fragrant dish is perfect for easy entertaining as it is all cooked in one pot.

1 onion, peeled and roughly chopped
2 red peppers, deseeded and cut into
   bite-sized pieces
3 large carrots, peeled and cut into
   bite-sized pieces
2 garlic cloves, peeled and chopped
1 tsp finely grated ginger
2 tsp ground cinnamon
1 tbsp dried mixed Mediterranean
   herbs, e.g. oregano, rosemary,
   thyme

1 x 400g/14oz can chopped tomatoes
2 tbsp artificial sweetener
600ml/1pt chicken stock made from
   Bovril
650g/1lb 7oz lean lamb, cubed
10 dried, ready-to-eat apricots, finely
   chopped
salt and freshly ground black pepper

to garnish:
chopped flat-leaf parsley

   Place the onions, peppers, carrots, garlic, ginger, cinnamon, dried herbs, tomatoes, sweetener and the stock in a large saucepan or casserole dish. Bring to the boil and then add the lamb. Bring back to the boil, cover tightly, reduce the heat and simmer gently for 1$^{1}/_{2}$ hours.

   Add the apricots and seasoning and cook for another 20–30 minutes or until the lamb is tender. Sprinkle the parsley over the stew and serve immediately.

**BONUS POINT**
The stew can be
frozen and stored
for up to a month
in the freezer.

# Sausage roast with celeriac mash

Mushrooms and sausages roasted with herbs and garlic are served with a rich gravy, perfectly complemented by a creamy mash.

**serves** 4
**preparation time**
30 minutes
**cooking time**
about 30 minutes
**syns per serving**
original **4½**
green **10½**
(using Bowyers
95% fat-free
sausages)

**4 onions, peeled and quartered**
**8–10 garlic cloves (with their skins**
**left on)**
**12 Bowyers 95% fat-free sausages**
**8 field or portobello mushrooms**
**3 tbsp white wine vinegar**
**2 tsp runny honey**
**1 tsp powdered mustard**
**4–5 sprigs of thyme**
**Fry Light for spraying**
**salt and freshly ground black pepper**

**for the 'mash':**
**750g/1lb 11oz celeriac, peeled and**
**roughly chopped**
**200g/7oz very low fat natural**
**fromage frais**
**2 tbsp chopped mixed herbs**
**salt and freshly ground black pepper**

**for the gravy:**
**1 small red onion, peeled and diced**
**400ml/14fl oz beef stock from Bovril**
**1 level tbsp cornflour**

Preheat the oven to 200°C/Gas 6. Place the onions, garlic, sausages and mushrooms in a large, non-stick roasting tray. Mix together the vinegar, honey and mustard and pour over and toss. Scatter over the sprigs of thyme, add seasoning and lightly spray with Fry Light. Place in the oven and bake for 25–30 minutes until the sausages are cooked.

Meanwhile, boil the celeriac in a pan of lightly salted water for 12–15 minutes or until tender. Drain, return to the pan and mash. Stir in the fromage frais and herbs, season and mix well. Set aside and keep warm.

To make the gravy, place the red onion in a pan with half the stock and bring to the boil. Reduce the heat and simmer for 5 minutes. Blend the cornflour with a little of the remaining stock and add to the pan with the rest of the stock. Season, bring to the boil and cook for a few minutes until thickened. Set aside and keep warm. To serve, divide the mash and the sausage mixture between four warmed plates and serve the gravy on the side. Accompany with green vegetables and carrots, if desired.

**BONUS POINT**
You can make the mash up to a few hours in advance. Just heat it up before serving.

**serves** 6–8
**preparation time**
20 minutes
**cooking time**
1–1½ hours
**syns per serving**
If serving 6:
original **½**
green **15½**
If serving 8:
original **½**
green **11½**

# Peppered roast beef with roasted root vegetables

The ultimate roast lunch, serve this succulent beef joint with a mixture of delicious roasted vegetables, which will please everyone at the table.

2 tbsp black peppercorns
1 tbsp dry mustard powder
1 tbsp dried mixed herbs
2 tsp sea salt
1 x 1.2kg/2lb 12oz lean beef sirloin
  joint (with all visible fat removed)

for the roasted vegetables:
500g/1lb 2oz celeriac, peeled and cut
into thick fingers

3 large carrots, peeled and cut into
thick fingers
400g/14oz swede, peeled and cut
into thick fingers
Fry Light for spraying
Salt and freshly ground black pepper

200ml/7fl oz beef stock made from
  Bovril
1 tbsp cornflour

ORIGINAL

■ Preheat the oven to 220°C/Gas 7. Place the peppercorns in a pestle and crush with a mortar until coarse. Mix with the dry mustard powder and dried herbs and sea salt. Rub the pepper mixture over the joint and place on a rack in a non-stick roasting tin. Roast the joint in the oven for 20 minutes, then reduce the oven temperature to 190°C/Gas 5 and cook for 30 minutes for rare; 45 minutes for medium or 1 hour for well done.

■ Meanwhile, cook the root vegetables in a large pan of boiling water for 15 minutes. Drain and place in a non-stick roasting tray. Spray with Fry Light, season well and cook for 20 minutes or until browned and tender.

**BONUS POINT**
You can ask your butcher to prepare and truss your beef joint for you, removing all the visible fat as he works.

■ When the joint is cooked to your liking, remove from the oven, cover with foil and set aside in a warm place to rest. Pour the stock into the roasting tin with the meat juices and bring to the boil over a high heat. Mix the cornflour with 2 tablespoons cold water, add to the gravy and whisk for 2–3 minutes until thickened. Strain into a jug and keep warm. To serve, carve the beef into thin slices and serve with the gravy and the roasted root vegetables.

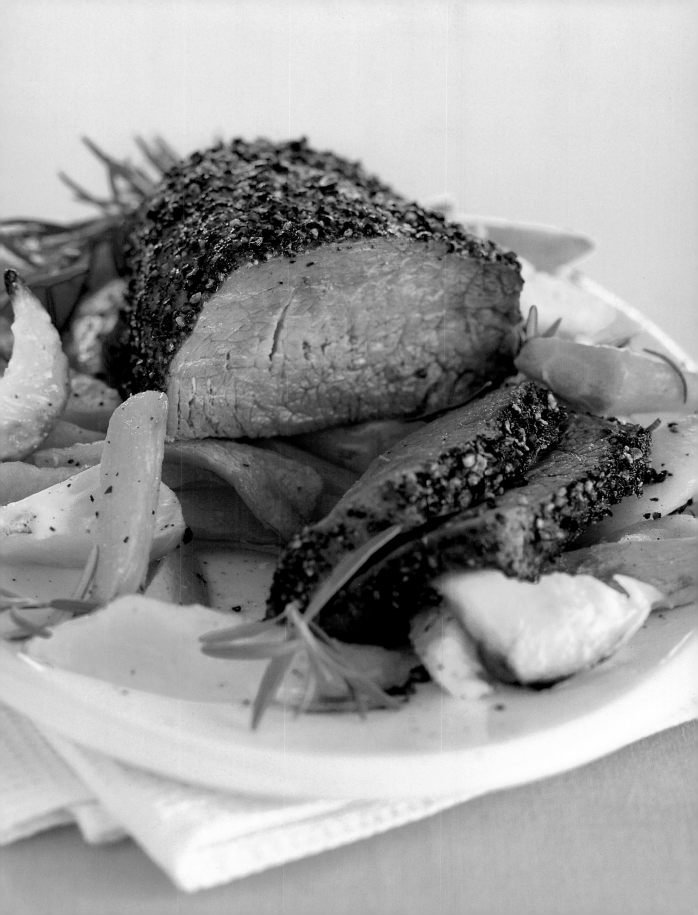

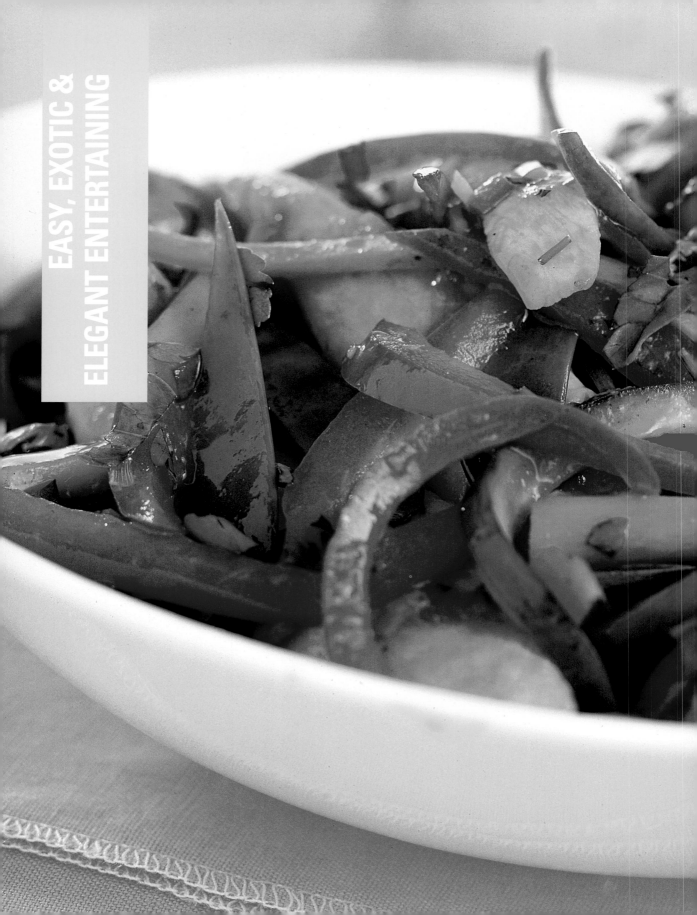

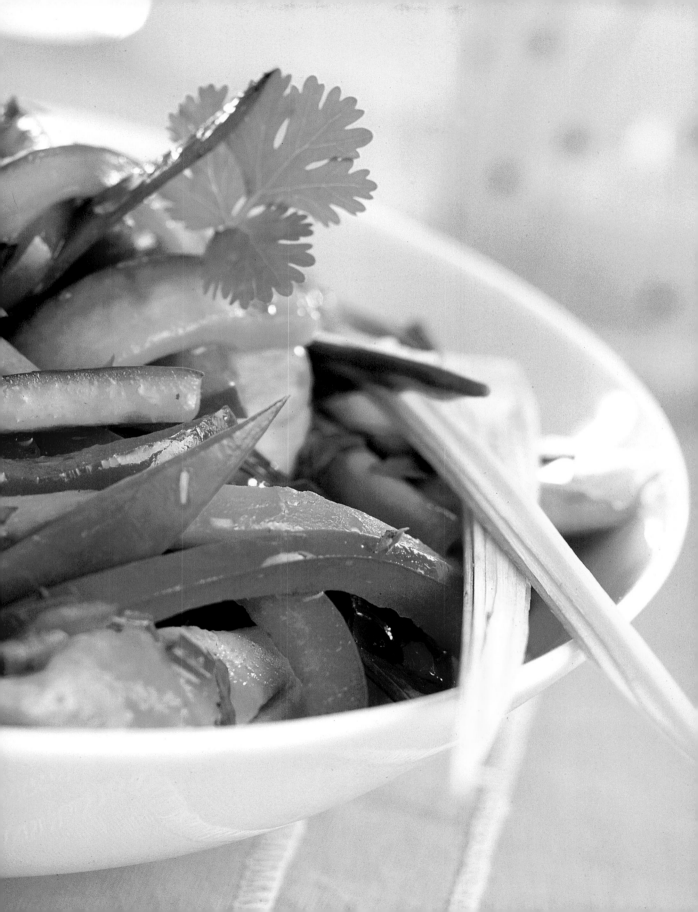

**serves** 4
**preparation time**
20 minutes
**cooking time**
about 15 minutes
**vegetarian**
**syns per serving**
original **18**
green **1/2**

GREEN

# Vegetable biriyani

Fragrant Basmati rice and a colourful medley of vegetables are cooked with Indian curry powder to create a rich, elegant and aromatic dish.

400g/14oz easy-cook Basmati rice
1 litre/1¾pt vegetable stock
3 tbsp mild curry powder
salt
1 onion, peeled and finely chopped
200g/7oz cauliflower florets
3 plum tomatoes, roughly chopped
1 courgette, diced

6 tbsp chopped coriander leaves
1 tbsp chopped mint leaves

to serve:
very low fat natural yogurt and a
    cucumber salad

■ Place the rice in a large, non-stick saucepan with the stock and the curry powder. Season with salt and bring to the boil. Cover, reduce the heat and simmer gently for 8–10 minutes.

■ Add the onion, cauliflower, tomatoes and courgette. Bring back to the boil, cover and cook over a low heat for 6–8 minutes or until the rice is cooked and tender and the stock is absorbed. Remove from the heat and let stand, covered, for 10 minutes.

■ Stir in the chopped herbs and serve immediately accompanied by yogurt and a cucumber salad.

**BONUS POINT**
This dish can be frozen for up to one month.

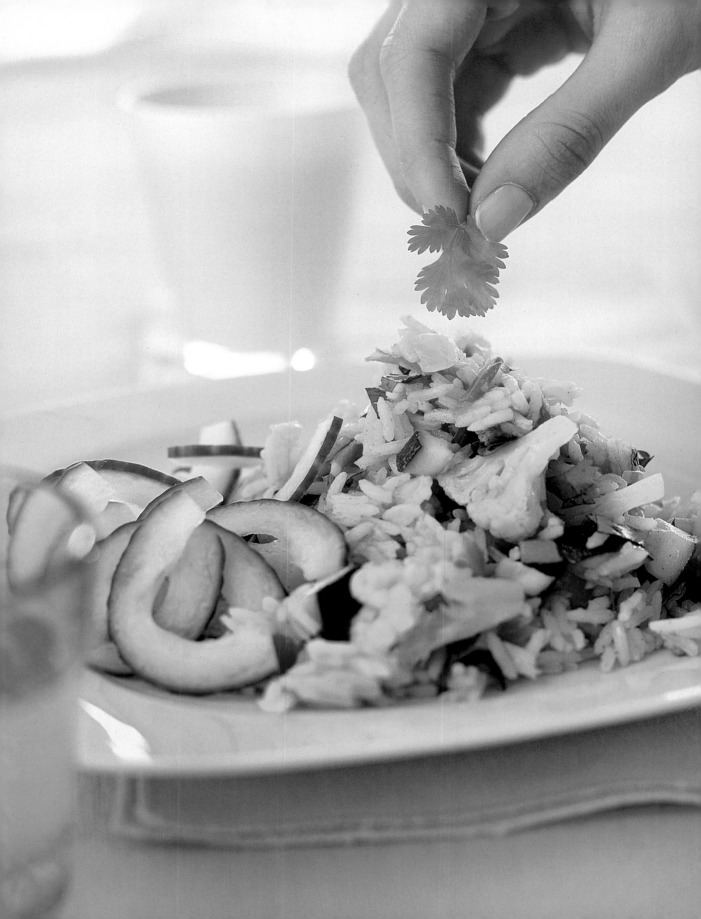

# Sicilian minted carrots and courgettes

**serves** 4
**preparation time**
5 minutes
**cooking time**
6–8 minutes
**vegetarian**
**syns per serving**
original **free**
green **free**

Serve with steamed rice and a flavoursome tomato salad, this simple but delicious dish is Free Food on Green and Original days.

3 carrots, peeled and cut into batons
400g/14oz courgettes, cut into
   batons
3 shallots, finely chopped
200ml/7fl oz chicken stock made
   from Bovril
3 tbsp chopped mint leaves

200g/7oz very low fat natural
   fromage frais
salt and freshly ground black pepper

to serve:
steamed rice
tomato salad

■ Place the carrots, courgettes and shallots in a large saucepan and add the stock. Cover and cook on a gentle heat, stirring occasionally, for 6–8 minutes or until the carrots and courgettes are just tender.

■ Sprinkle over the chopped mint and stir in the fromage frais. Season and toss to mix well. Serve immediately accompanied by steamed rice (on an Original day, this counts as 2 Syns per 30g/1oz cooked weight) and a tomato salad.

**BONUS POINT**
The salad is equally delicious served on a bed of soft noodles.

# Minted asparagus risotto

This Italian-style rice dish requires very little from the cook, except stirring. When entertaining, garnish with wild rocket leaves.

**serves** 4
**preparation time**
15 minutes
**cooking time**
35 minutes
**vegetarian**
**syns per serving**
original **12**
green **½**

Fry Light for spraying
1 red onion, peeled and finely
   chopped
2 garlic cloves, peeled and finely
   chopped
250g/9oz arborio or risotto rice

900ml/1½pt boiling hot vegetable
   stock
400g/14oz asparagus tips, trimmed
3 tbsp finely chopped mint leaves
3 tbsp finely chopped flat-leaf parsley
salt and freshly ground black pepper
1 level tbsp grated Parmesan cheese

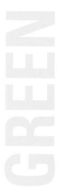

GREEN

■ Spray a large, non-stick saucepan with Fry Light and place over a medium heat. Add the onion and stir-fry for 3–4 minutes. Add the garlic and the rice and stir-fry for 2–3 minutes.

■ Add a large ladleful of the boiling hot stock and stir continuously until the stock has been absorbed. Repeat adding ladlefuls and allowing to absorb until half the stock is used up and then add the asparagus tips.

■ Continue to cook in this manner, stirring constantly, until all the stock has been used. The whole process should take about 20–25 minutes.

■ When all the stock has been absorbed and the rice is creamy and al dente (tender, but still retaining a bite), remove from the heat and stir in the chopped herbs. Season well and serve in warmed plates or bowls, sprinkled with the grated cheese.

**BONUS POINT**
Always keep the stock boiling hot when making the risotto.

**serves** 4
**preparation time**
20 minutes
**cooking time**
20–25 minutes
**syns per serving**
original **1½**
green **19**

# Luxury seafood cakes with fennel salad

These colourful and flavoursome fish cakes are complemented perfectly with the delicate slices of fresh fennel and cucumber salad.

700g/1lb 9oz salmon fillet, cut into
   cubes
250g/9oz raw tiger prawns, shelled
1 tsp finely grated garlic
1 tsp finely grated ginger
2 level tbsp reduced calorie
   mayonnaise
1 red pepper, deseeded and very
   finely chopped
4 tbsp chopped mixed herbs,
   e.g. dill, chives, parsley

6 spring onions, very finely sliced
salt and freshly ground black pepper
Fry Light for spraying

for the salad:
2 large bulbs fennel, trimmed,
   quartered and thinly sliced
1 cucumber, thinly sliced with a
   vegetable peeler
juice of 2 lemons
salt and freshly ground black pepper

■ Place the salmon and prawns in a food processor with the garlic, ginger and mayonnaise. Blend until fairly smooth and then transfer to a bowl. Stir in the red pepper, chopped herbs and spring onions. Season, cover and chill overnight.

■ Divide the mixture into 16 portions and shape each one into a ball.

■ Preheat the oven to 200°C/Gas 6 and line a baking sheet with baking parchment and lightly spray with Fry Light. Place the 'cakes' on the baking sheet and bake for 20–25 minutes or until cooked through and golden. Set aside and keep warm.

■ Make the salad by mixing together all the ingredients. Season well. To serve, place four seafood 'cakes' on each serving plate and accompany with the fennel salad.

**BONUS POINT**
The cakes can be frozen once made, but only if the fish used in them is fresh and not previously frozen.

ORIGINAL

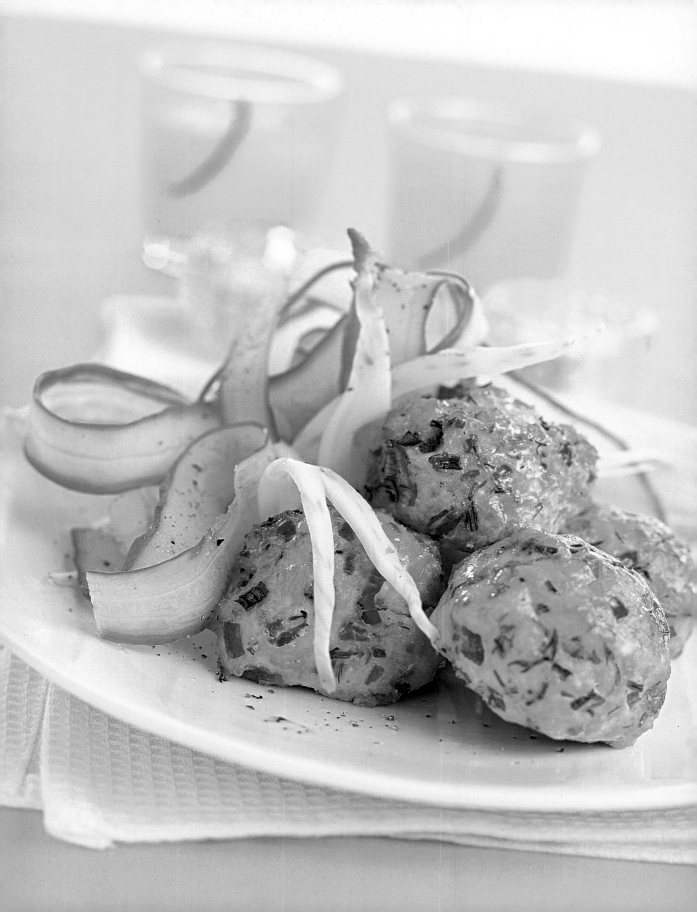

**serves** 4
**preparation time**
25 minutes
**cooking time**
about 15 minutes
**syns per serving**
original **1**
green **6**

ORIGINAL

# Herbed grilled mussels with radicchio

Easy and quick to prepare, these tasty mussels are prepared with fresh and flavoursome ingredients.

2 litres/3½pt fresh 'live' mussels
bay leaf
200ml/7fl oz vegetable stock
2 slices of Nimble wholemeal bread
3 garlic cloves, peeled and very finely
   chopped
3 plum tomatoes, deseeded and very
   finely chopped
2 shallots, very finely chopped

2 tbsp finely chopped flat-leaf parsley
1 tbsp finely snipped chives
1 tbsp finely chopped basil
1 tbsp finely grated lemon zest
juice of 1 lemon
salt and freshly ground black pepper
Fry Light for spraying
2 heads of radicchio or endive

Rinse the mussels under cold running water and scrub to remove any 'beards' or barnacles. Discard any that are open and place the mussels in a large saucepan with the bay leaf and stock. Cover and bring to the boil, shaking the pan occasionally, and cook for 4–5 minutes or until all the mussels have opened. Discard any that have remained closed. Drain the mussels and remove the top shell of each one, leaving you with a mussel in each half shell. Place the mussels on a large baking tray, in a single layer.

Whizz the bread in a food processor to give you breadcrumbs and transfer to a bowl with the garlic, tomatoes and shallots. Stir in the chopped herbs, lemon zest and juice. Season and stir to mix well. Spoon this mixture between the mussels in their shells, spray with Fry Light and place under a medium grill (about 10cm/4in away from the heat source) for 6–8 minutes or until lightly golden.

Separate the leaves of the radicchio or endive, wash and spin dry and arrange on four serving plates. Divide the mussels between them and serve immediately.

**BONUS POINT**
Any mussels that are open before cooking or closed after cooking are unhealthy so it is important that you discard them.

# Seared squid with tomato salad

Quickly cooked in a really hot pan, juicy and tender squid is tossed with an oriental-inspired dressing and served on salad leaves.

**serves** 4
**preparation time**
20 minutes
**cooking time**
6–8 minutes
**syns per serving**
original **free**
green **4¹/₂**

1 tsp finely grated ginger
2 tsp finely grated garlic
1 tbsp finely grated lemon zest
1 tbsp finely grated orange zest
1 red chilli, deseeded and chopped
4 tbsp light soy sauce
1 tbsp fish sauce
2 tbsp artificial sweetener
1 tbsp finely chopped lemongrass

2 tbsp finely chopped coriander leaves
juice of 2 lemons
500g/1lb 2oz squid tubes
2 plum tomatoes, deseeded and roughly chopped
¹/₂ small iceberg lettuce, shredded
a large handful of mint leaves, roughly torn

■ In a large mixing bowl, mix together the ginger, garlic, lemon and orange zest, red chilli, soy sauce, fish sauce, sweetener, lemongrass, coriander leaves and lemon juice. Set aside for 20 minutes for the flavours to develop.

■ Wash the squid, clean and cut into bite-sized pieces. Lightly score the flesh in a criss-cross pattern with a small, sharp knife and pat the pieces dry on kitchen paper.

■ Heat a large, non-stick frying pan over a high heat and, when very hot, add the squid in batches (do not overcrowd) and cook for 1–2 minutes. Transfer to the bowl containing the ginger-garlic mixture and toss to mix.

■ Mix together the tomatoes, shredded lettuce and mint leaves and divide between four serving plates. Top each serving with the squid mixture, check the seasoning and serve immediately.

**ORIGINAL**

**BONUS POINT**
Never overcook squid as it will become rubbery and tough.

181

**serves** 4
**preparation time**
15 minutes
**cooking time**
about 5 minutes
**syns per serving**
original **1**
green **3**

ORIGINAL

# Herb, chilli and garlic sautéed prawns on vegetable spaghetti

Almost Free on an Original day, this stunning and really delicious dish is perfect for easy entertaining.

for the 'spaghetti':
3 carrots, peeled and trimmed
3 courgettes, trimmed
salt and freshly ground black pepper

2 tsp olive oil
28–30 raw, large tiger prawns, shelled
(leaving the tails on)
1 red chilli, deseeded and finely

sliced
4 garlic cloves, peeled and very thin-ly
sliced
juice and finely grated zest of
1 lemon
4 tbsp finely chopped flat-leaf parsley

■ Using a mandolin or a serrated vegetable peeler, carefully cut the carrots and courgettes into thin, long strands (to resemble spaghetti). Bring a large pan of lightly salted water to the boil and add the vegetable strips. Cook for 2–3 minutes, drain and keep warm.

■ Heat the oil in a large, non-stick frying pan and when hot add the prawns, chilli, garlic, lemon zest and juice. Stir-fry on a high heat for 3–4 minutes or until the prawns turn pink and are cooked through. Stir in the chopped parsley, season and remove from the heat.

■ To serve, divide the warm, drained carrot and courgette 'spaghetti' between four warmed bowls or plates and top with the cooked prawns. Spoon over any pan juices and serve immediately.

**BONUS POINT**
You could substitute small cubes of salmon for the prawns if desired.

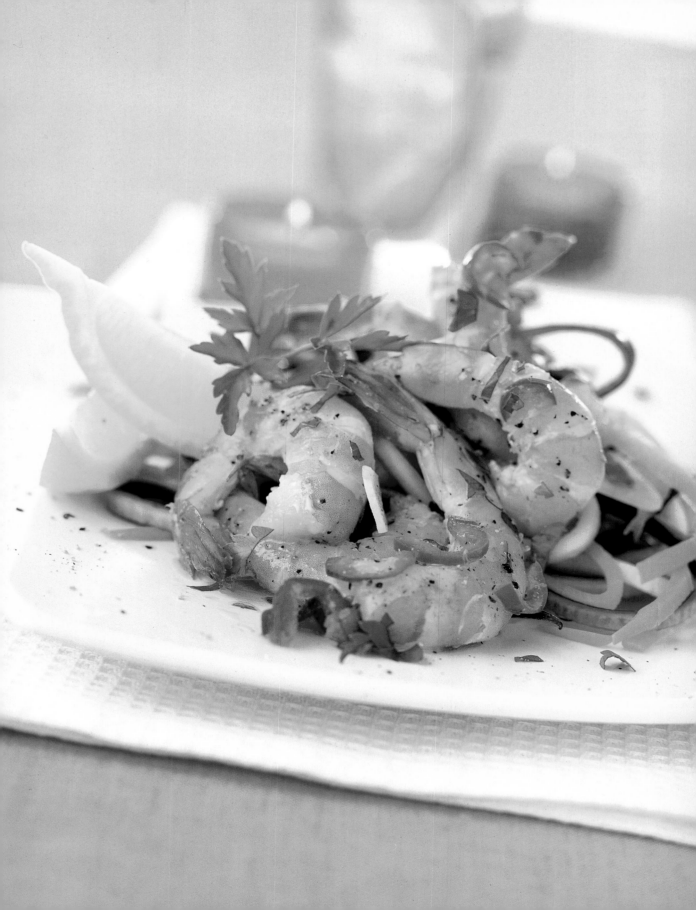

**serves** 4
**preparation time**
15 minutes
**cooking time**
25 minutes
**syns per serving**
original **free**
green **8**

ORIGINAL

# Grilled Mediterranean chicken

Sweet yellow and red peppers, ripe tomatoes and smoked paprika bring the flavours of the Mediterranean to this succulent and tender chicken.

4 skinless, boneless chicken breasts
Fry Light for spraying
1 onion, peeled and finely sliced
3 garlic cloves, peeled and crushed
1 red pepper, deseeded and thinly sliced
1 yellow pepper, deseeded and finely sliced
1 x 400g/14oz can chopped tomatoes with herbs
150ml/¼pt chicken stock made with Bovril

1 tbsp sweet paprika
salt and freshly ground black pepper
1 romaine lettuce, washed and torn into large pieces
juice of 1 lemon
2 tbsp very low fat natural yogurt
2 anchovies, crushed

to garnish:
chopped flat-leaf parsley

■ Cut the chicken into thin strips. Lightly spray a ridged griddle pan with Fry Light and place over a high heat. Add the chicken and fry for 2–3 minutes on each side until sealed.

■ Place the onion, garlic, peppers and tomatoes in a saucepan and bring to the boil. Add the stock and paprika and the chicken and cook over a medium heat for 10–15 minutes until the chicken is cooked through. Season well.

■ To assemble the salad, place the lettuce in a large bowl. In a separate small bowl mix together the lemon juice and yogurt. Season and add to the salad leaves together with the crushed anchovies. Toss to mix well and serve with the chicken.  Garnish with the chopped flat-leaf parsley.

**BONUS POINT**
For a change, use strips of turkey instead of chicken.

# Japanese chicken teriyaki skewers

Here succulent chicken breasts are cubed and marinated in Japanese seasonings and then grilled to perfection.

**serves** 4
**preparation time**
15 minutes +
4–5 hours
marinating
**cooking time**
12 minutes
**syns per serving**
original **2**
green **13**

**6 large chicken breast fillets, skinned**

**for the marinade:**
**2 tbsp clear honey**
**2 tsp ground ginger**
**1 tsp garlic salt**
**2 tbsp mirin or rice wine vinegar**
**a few drops of sesame oil**
**juice of 1 orange**
**$1/2$ tsp ground cinnamon**
**5 tbsp light soy sauce**

**for the skewers:**
**8 spring onions**
**freshly ground black pepper**
**Fry Light for spraying**

Cut the chicken breasts into bite-sized pieces and place in a large mixing bowl.

Mix together all the marinade ingredients, pour over the chicken and mix well to coat evenly. Cover and marinate in the fridge for 4–5 hours, or overnight if time permits.

Cut the spring onions into 6cm/$2^1/4$in lengths. Remove the chicken from the marinade and thread alternately with the spring onions on eight pre-soaked bamboo or metal skewers.

Preheat a grill to medium-high. Spray a grill rack with Fry Light and place the skewers on it. Lightly spray them with Fry Light and cook under the grill for 5–6 minutes on each side or until just cooked through and browned. Serve immediately.

**BONUS POINT**
You could make slashes in each chicken breast and marinate as above and then bake in the oven.

185

# Thai-style aromatic chicken stir-fry

ORIGINAL

This quick and flavour-packed stir-fry of tender chicken strips and vegetables is best cooked moments before you sit down to eat.

Fry Light for spraying
4 chicken breasts (skinned and boned), cut into thin strips
2 tbsp very finely chopped lemongrass
1 tsp finely grated fresh root ginger
2 garlic cloves, peeled and crushed
1 red chilli, deseeded and finely chopped
2–3 lime leaves, very finely shredded (optional)
juice and finely grated zest of 1 lime
1 red pepper, deseeded and cut into thin strips
100g/3½ oz mangetout, halved lengthways

1 cucumber, deseeded and cut into thin strips
1 carrot, peeled and cut into thin strips
90ml/3fl oz chicken stock made from Bovril
3 tbsp soy sauce
1 tbsp sweet chilli sauce
a small handful of chopped coriander leaves

to serve:
pak-choi or cabbage

■ Spray a large, non-stick wok or frying pan with Fry Light and heat until hot. Add the chicken and stir-fry over a high heat for 4–5 minutes, until just cooked through. Then remove with a slotted spoon and keep warm.

■ Re-spray the pan with Fry Light and when hot, add the lemongrass, ginger, garlic, chilli, lime leaves, lime zest and juice, red pepper, mangetout, cucumber and carrot. Stir-fry over a high heat for 3–4 minutes and then return the chicken to the pan with the stock and soy sauce. Cook for 2–3 minutes and then stir in the chilli sauce and scatter over the coriander leaves. Serve immediately, with pak-choi or cabbage.

**BONUS POINT**
For a Free Food meal on a Green day, omit the chicken and replace with some more vegetables.

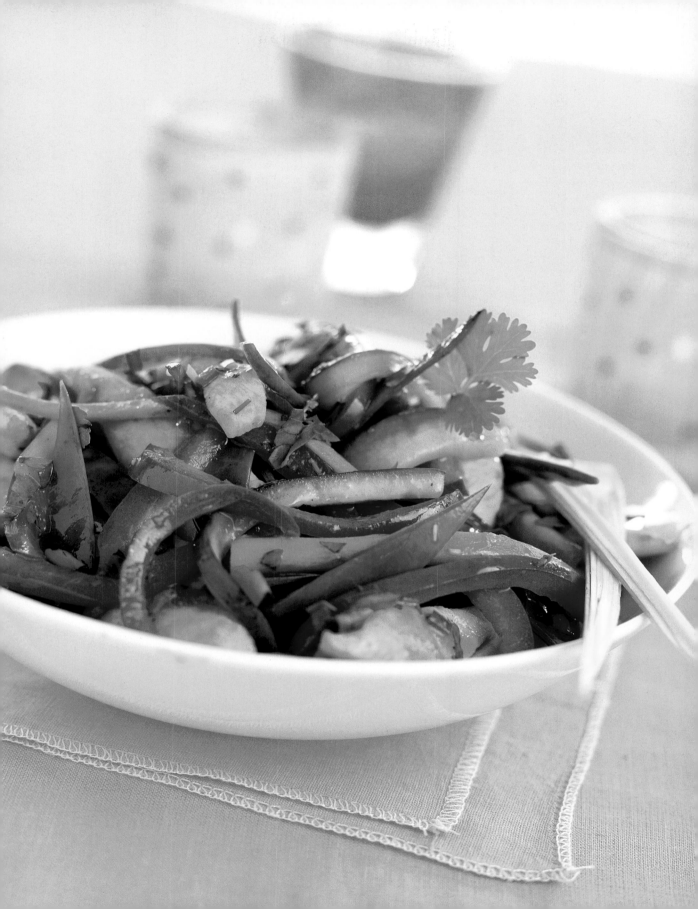

**serves** 4
**preparation time**
20 minutes
**cooking time**
about 30 minutes
**vegetarian**
**syns per serving**
original **11**
green **free**

GREEN

# Middle Eastern vegetable casserole with couscous

Vegetables and chickpeas are cooked slowly with subtle Moroccan-style spices and herbs in this warming supper dish.

1 tsp finely grated ginger
2 tsp ground cumin
1 tsp garlic salt
$1/2$ tsp sweet smoked paprika
2 red onions, peeled and quartered
2 carrots, peeled and roughly chopped
1 courgette, halved lengthways and roughly chopped
1 medium aubergine, cut into bite-sized pieces
1 red pepper, deseeded and roughly chopped

1 x 400g/14oz can chopped tomatoes
2–3 tbsp artificial sweetener
400ml/14fl oz vegetable stock
1 x 200g/7oz can chickpeas, drained
salt and freshly ground black pepper
175g/6oz dried couscous
4 spring onions, finely chopped
2 tbsp finely chopped red pepper

to serve:
a large bunch of coriander leaves, roughly chopped

■ Preheat the oven to 200°C/Gas 6. Place the ginger, cumin, garlic salt, paprika, red onions, carrots, courgette, aubergine, red pepper, tomatoes, sweetener, stock and chickpeas in a flame- and ovenproof casserole dish (with a tight-fitting lid). Place over a high heat and bring the mixture to the boil. Season well, cover tightly and cook in the oven for 20–25 minutes.

■ Meanwhile, place the couscous, spring onions and red pepper in a bowl. Season and pour over about 300ml/$1/2$pt boiling water to just cover. Cover tightly and let sit undisturbed for 15–20 minutes.

■ To serve, remove the casserole from the oven, sprinkle over the chopped coriander and ladle into warmed, shallow bowls. Fluff up the grains of couscous with a fork and serve with the casserole.

**BONUS POINT**
Try serving the vegetable mixture with plain steamed rice.

# Calypso lamb steaks with Cajun tomato and red pepper sauce

This Caribbean-inspired dish is a really tasty way to serve lamb steaks – grilled and accompanied by a fresh tomato sauce.

8 lean lamb steaks
2 tsp ground allspice
4 tsp Cajun spice mix
salt
Fry Light for spraying
1 red onion, peeled and finely
   chopped
2 garlic cloves, peeled and finely
   chopped
1 tsp ground cumin
2 red peppers, deseeded and finely
   chopped
1 x 400g/14oz can chopped tomatoes

1 tbsp thyme leaves
3 tbsp chopped parsley
salt and freshly ground black pepper

**serves** 4
**preparation time**
10 minutes
**cooking time**
about 20 minutes
**syns per serving**
original **free**
green **22**

■ Rub the lamb steaks with the ground allspice and half the Cajun spice mix. Season and place on a grill rack under a preheated medium-hot grill for 4–5 minutes on each side, or according to taste.

■ Meanwhile, lightly spray a non-stick pan with Fry light and add the onions, garlic and cumin. Stir-fry over a medium heat for 2–3 minutes and then add the remaining Cajun spice mix, the peppers and tomatoes and bring to the boil. Turn down the heat and simmer, stirring occasionally, for about 5 minutes. Stir in the chopped herbs and season well.

■ To serve, place two grilled steaks on warmed serving plates and spoon the sauce around.

**BONUS POINT**
For a smoother sauce, use a passata with herbs instead of the chopped tomatoes.

ORIGINAL

189

**serves** 4
**preparation time**
10 minutes +
4–5 hours
marinating
**cooking time**
10–12 minutes
**syns per serving**
original **1¹/₂**
green **12¹/₂**

# Griddled Tunisian lamb with tzatziki

This lamb, marinated with Tunisian spices and seasonings, is quickly cooked in a grill pan and served with a cool and minty dip.

2 tsp ground cumin

1 tsp ground cinnamon

2 tsp paprika

¹/₄ tsp ground cardamom

¹/₄ tsp ground cloves

3 garlic cloves, peeled and crushed

4 tbsp white wine vinegar

200g/7oz very low fat natural
   yogurt

2 tbsp clear honey

salt and freshly ground black pepper

4 lean lamb chops or steaks
   (trimmed of any visible fat)

for the tzatziki:

1 large cucumber

3 spring onions, finely chopped

250g/8oz very low fat natural
   yogurt

¹/₄ tsp ground cumin

3 tbsp finely chopped mint leaves

1 tsp artificial sweetener

Mix together the cumin, cinnamon, paprika, cardamom, cloves, garlic, vinegar, yogurt and honey. Add seasoning.

Place the lamb in a shallow mixing bowl and pour over the spice mixture. Toss to coat well, cover and marinate in the fridge for 4–5 hours, or overnight if time permits.

Meanwhile, make the tzatziki. Halve the cucumber lengthways and, using a small teaspoon, remove the seeds. Finely dice the cucumber flesh and place in a bowl with the remaining ingredients and stir to mix well. Season, cover and chill until ready to serve.

Heat a ridged griddle pan over a high heat and when hot add the marinated lamb and cook for 5–6 minutes on each side until just cooked through and tender. Check the seasoning and serve on warmed plates accompanied by the tzatziki.

**BONUS POINT**
If time permits, try to marinate the meat for 24 hours for a really tender result.

190

# Moroccan pork kofta tagine

If served with salad or steamed vegetables, this hearty dish of meatballs in a fragrant Middle Eastern-style sauce is perfect when entertaining.

**serves** 4
**preparation time**
20 minutes
**cooking time**
16–18 minutes
**syns per serving**
original **free**
green **12**

900g/2lb very lean minced pork
2 red onions, peeled and very finely
   chopped
2 garlic cloves, peeled and crushed
1 tsp ground ginger
2 tbsp ground cumin
1 tbsp ground coriander
4–5 tbsp chopped coriander leaves
3–4 tbsp chopped mint leaves
salt and freshly ground black pepper
$1/2$ tsp sweet paprika or cayenne

$1/2$ tsp ground cinnamon
finely grated zest and juice of
   1 lemon
500ml/16fl oz chicken stock made
   from Bovril

**to serve:**
couscous, rice or salad
chopped mint leaves
chopped coriander leaves

■ Place the mince in a large mixing bowl with half the onion, all the garlic and ginger, half the cumin and half the ground coriander. Add the chopped herbs and season well. Mix thoroughly using your fingers and shape the mixture into walnut-size balls. Set aside.

■ Place the remaining onion in a non-stick frying pan with the remaining spices, the paprika and the lemon zest and juice and stock. Bring to the boil and add the koftas, turn the heat to medium-low, cover and cook for 12–15 minutes, stirring occasionally, until cooked through and tender. Season and serve immediately with couscous or rice (on an Original day, these count as 2 Syns per 30g/1oz cooked weight) and salad, garnished with chopped mint and coriander.

ORIGINAL

**BONUS POINT**
Try using lean chicken or beef mince instead of the pork. This dish freezes well for up to a month.

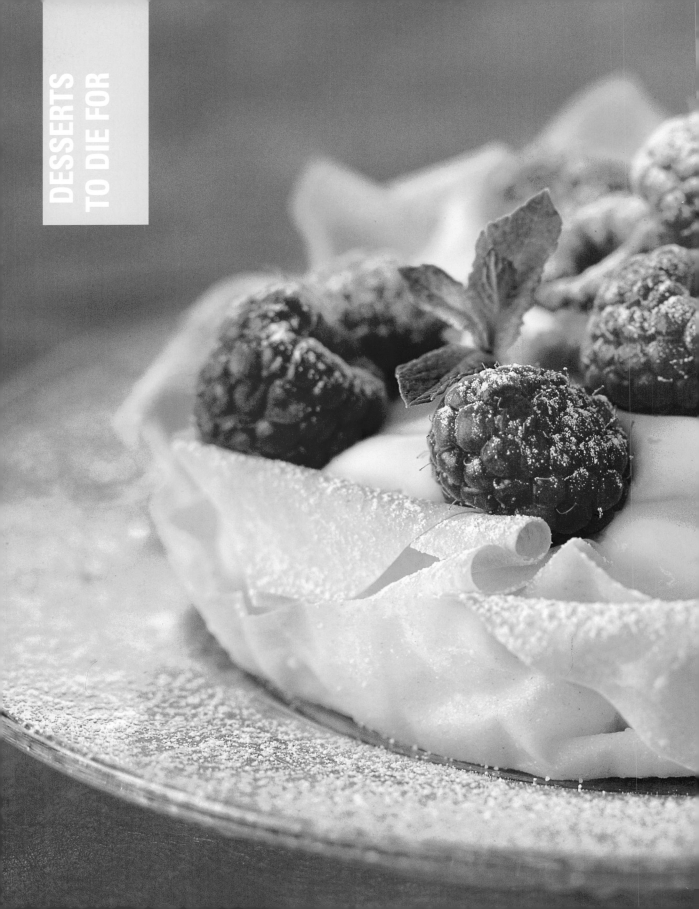

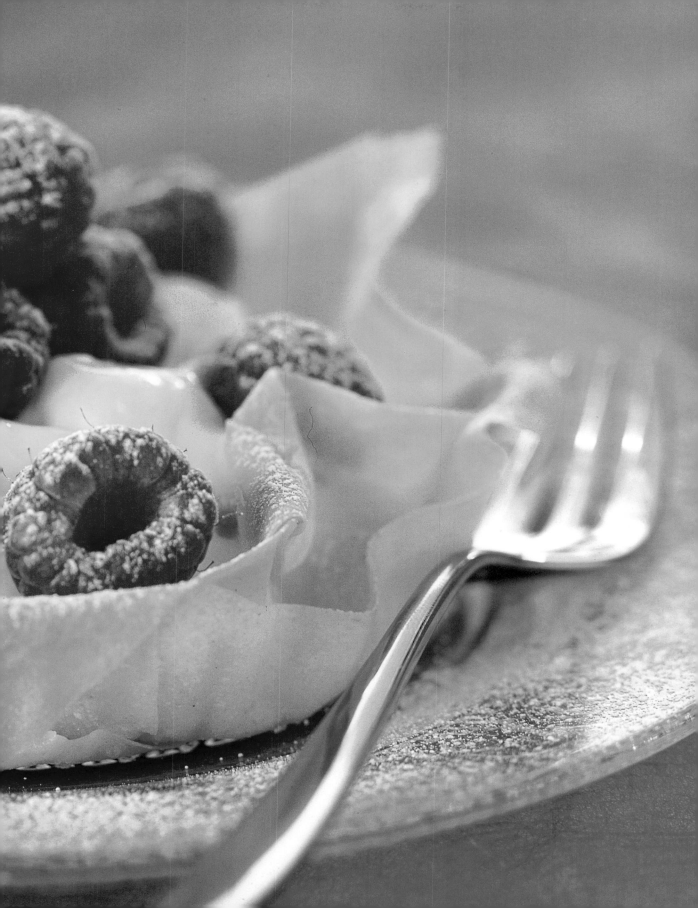

**serves** 4
**preparation time**
20 minutes +
chilling
**vegetarian**
**syns per serving**
original **3**
green **3**

# Berry **jelly** trifles

This satisfying pudding combines jelly, sponge fingers and fresh fruit and will certainly be popular with all the family.

1 pack Rowntrees' sugar-free
   strawberry jelly crystals
6 sponge fingers
2 tbsp sweet sherry
2 tbsp apple juice
400g/14oz Müllerlight strawberry-
   flavoured yogurt
4 tbsp very low fat natural fromage
   frais
300g/10oz mixed summer berries
1 level tsp icing sugar

to garnish:
mint leaves
chopped jelly

■  Prepare the jelly according to the packet instructions and then pour into a shallow, non-stick Swiss-roll tin. Cover the tin and chill in the fridge until set.

■  Roughly break up the sponge fingers and place in the bottom of four wide dessert bowls. Sprinkle over the sherry and apple juice.

■  Roughly chop the jelly into cubes (reserving a little bit for the garnish) and spoon over the soaked sponge fingers.

■  Spoon the strawberry yogurt over the jelly and top with a tablespoon of the fromage frais on each serving. Scatter the berries over the fromage frais, lightly dust with icing sugar and serve garnished with mint leaves and the remaining chopped jelly.

GREEN/ORIGINAL

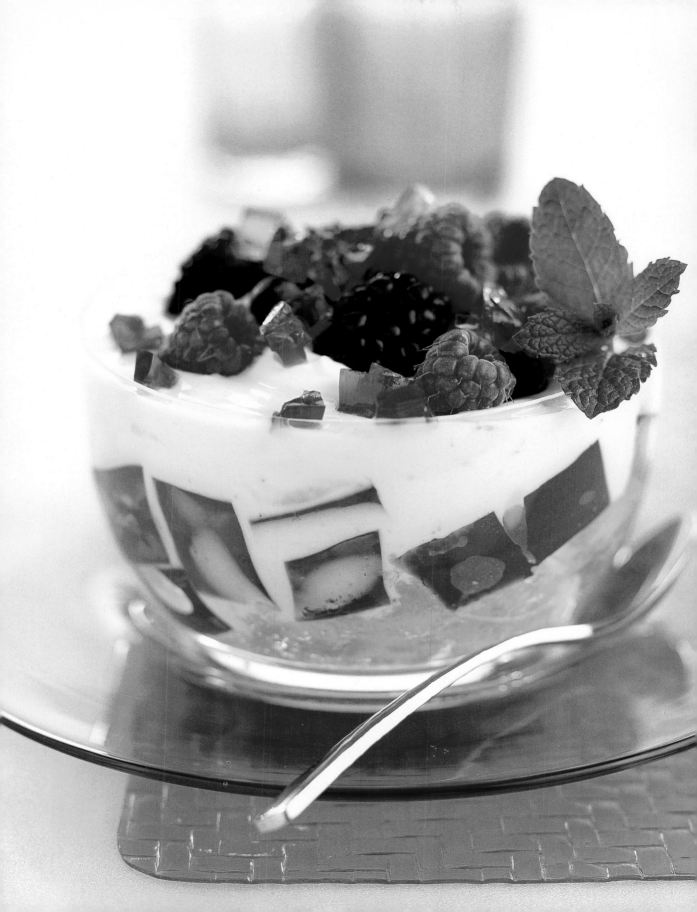

serves 4
preparation time
5 minutes +
chilling
vegetarian
syns per serving
original **4¹/₂**
green **4¹/₂**

# Pear, orange and toffee pots

A truly satisfying combination of fresh pears layered with oranges, toffee yogurt and crunchy gingernut biscuits.

5 dessert pears
2 tsp finely grated orange zest
1 tbsp orange juice
2 tbsp artificial sweetener
2 x 200g/7oz Müllerlight toffee-
   flavoured yogurt

2 oranges, peeled and segmented
4 tbsp very low fat natural fromage
   frais
2 gingernut biscuits, coarsely
crushed

Peel the pears and then core and roughly chop them. Place in a saucepan with the orange zest, juice, sweetener and 4 tablespoons of water. Cook over a medium heat for 4–5 minutes until the pears are just tender.

To serve, layer the pear mixture, toffee yogurt and orange segments in four dessert glasses. Top each serving with a tablespoon of fromage frais and sprinkle over the crushed biscuits. Chill for 1–2 hours before serving.

**BONUS POINT**
When preparing pears and apples, have a bowl of water with added lemon juice to hand. As you chop the fruit, drop it into the lemon water to prevent discoloration.

GREEN/ORIGINAL

# Chocolate and caramel cheesecakes

You can have your cake and eat it with these delicious low fat cheese-cakes topped with a drizzle of caramel.

serves 4
**preparation time**
about 20 minutes
+ chilling
**vegetarian**
**syns per serving**
original **6¹/2**
green **6¹/2**

6 gingernut biscuits
1 level tbsp low fat spread, melted
Fry Light for spraying
2 x 200g/7oz pot Müllerlight
    chocolate-flavoured yogurt
a few drops of vanilla essence

2 sachets gelatine
cocoa powder (optional)

for the caramel:
2 tbsp granulated sugar
2 tbsp water

■ Put the biscuits in a processor and blend until finely crumbed. Place in a bowl and add the melted spread and a couple of sprays of Fry Light.

■ Line a non-stick baking sheet with non-stick baking parchment and place four individual pastry rings (about 7–8cm/2³/4–3¹/4in in diameter) on it. Divide and spoon the biscuit mixture into the rings, pressing down well with the back of a spoon. Chill in the fridge.

■ Place the chocolate yogurt and vanilla in a bowl and set aside.

■ Dissolve the gelatine in 4–5 tbsp of water in another bowl over a pan of gently simmering water. When dissolved, stir thoroughly into the chocolate mixture. Spoon this over the biscuit bases and return to the fridge for 4–5 hours or until set. Run a sharp knife around the inside of each ring and place on individual serving plates.

■ Before serving, place the sugar and water in a small, clean saucepan and heat gently until the mixture starts to caramelise. Take off the heat and quickly drizzle over the four cheesecakes. Lightly dust with cocoa (if using) and serve immediately.

**BONUS POINT**
The cheesecakes can be prepared up to a day before and kept in the fridge. You then only need to make the caramel.

GREEN/ORIGINAL

GREEN/ORIGINAL

serves 4
**preparation time**
15 minutes
**cooking time**
5–6 minutes
**vegetarian**
**syns per serving**
original **3**
green **3**

# Mango and cardamom brulée

In this scrumptious dessert, yogurt flavoured with cardamom seeds and vanilla blanket juicy ripe mangoes.

**3 large, ripe mangoes**
**2 x 150g/5oz pots Total Greek 0%**
  **fat natural yogurt**
**2–3 cardamom pods**
**a few drops vanilla essence**
**3–4 tbsp artificial sweetener**
**4 tbsp caster sugar**

**to serve:**
**mango slices**

▢ Peel, stone and finely chop the mango flesh and set aside.

▢ Place the yogurt in a mixing bowl. Peel the skin from the cardamom pods and carefully remove the small black seeds. Place the seeds in a mortar and crush with the pestle until fine. Alternatively, place them on a board and crush with a rolling pin. Stir into the yogurt with the vanilla and sweetener.

▢ Divide the chopped mango between four individual glass ramekins and top with the yogurt mixture. Sprinkle over the caster sugar.

▢ Heat a grill to medium-high. Place the ramekins on a rack under the grill for 5–6 minutes until the top is golden and slightly caramelised. Be careful to cool before serving and then serve with a layer of mango slices arranged over the top of each ramekin.

**BONUS POINT**
Use any selection of fruit, e.g. strawberries, blackcurrants or grapes, to vary this easy dessert.

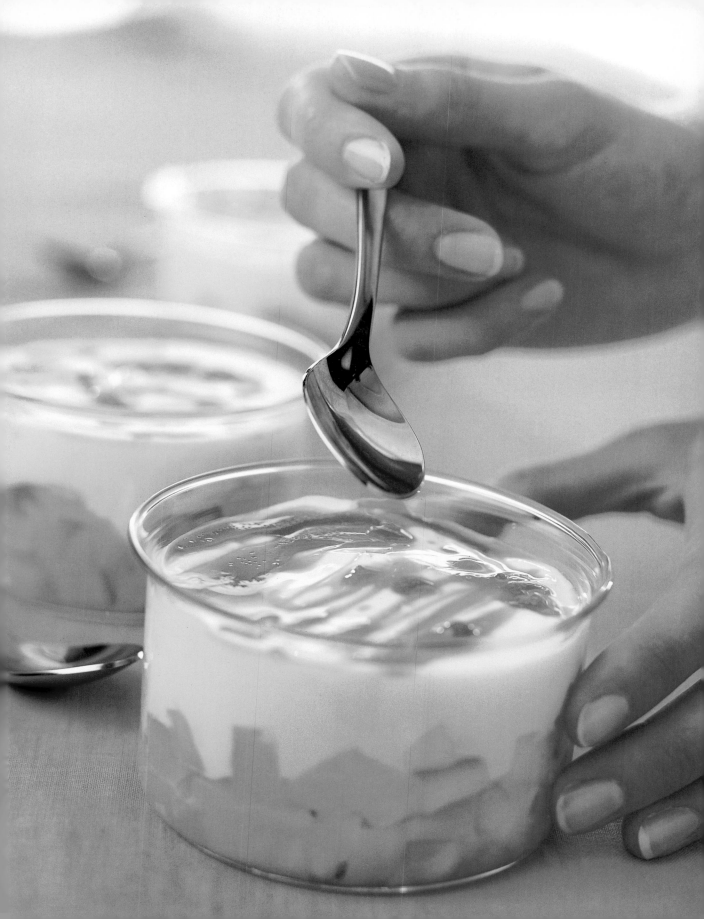

serves **4**
**preparation time**
20 minutes +
sultana soaking
time + freezing
**vegetarian**
**syns per serving**
original **4**
green **4**

# Golden sultana and Armagnac ice cream

A great freezer standby for last-minute entertaining, this rich and boozy ice cream is definitely not one for the kids.

**30g/1oz golden sultanas**
**4 tbsp Armagnac**
**200g/7oz low fat custard**
**300g/10oz Müllerlight vanilla-**
 **flavoured yogurt**
**a few drops vanilla essence**

**to garnish:**
**mint leaves**

In a small bowl place the sultanas and pour over the Armagnac. Cover and leave to stand for 3–4 hours.

In a large bowl, mix together the custard, vanilla yogurt and vanilla essence. Add the soaked sultanas and stir to mix well.

Pour the mixture into a shallow freezerproof container, cover and place in the freezer. Freeze for 4–5 hours, but stirring the mixture with a fork every 30 minutes to break up any ice crystals. Then return to the freezer and freeze for a further 2 hours or until firm.

Before serving, remove the ice cream from the freezer and stand at room temperature for about 20 minutes or until soft enough to scoop. Serve, scooped into chilled bowls and garnished with mint leaves.

**BONUS POINT**
Use cognac as an alternative to the Armagnac, or even dark rum, if desired.

GREEN/ORIGINAL

200

# Strawberry and meringue 'sandwiches'

These pretty puddings, where chewy and crispy meringue is partnered with fruity yogurt, can be quickly assembled to great effect.

**serves** 4
**preparation time**
15 minutes
**cooking time**
about 40 minutes
**vegetarian**
**syns per serving**
original **2¹/₂**
green **2¹/₂**

2 small egg whites
35g/1½ oz golden caster sugar
1 tsp raspberry vinegar
100g/3½ oz Müllerlight vanilla-
   flavoured yogurt
100g/3½ oz strawberries, hulled and
   roughly chopped

to serve:
cocoa powder and icing sugar
   (optional)
mint leaves

■ Preheat the oven to 150°C/Gas 2.

■ Line two large, non-stick baking sheets with non-stick baking parchment. Whisk the egg whites until peaked and then gradually whisk in the sugar and the raspberry vinegar until stiff and glossy. Spoon or pipe the mixture onto the prepared sheets to give you eight circles, roughly 4–5cm/1³/₄–2in in diameter. Bake in the oven for 35–40 minutes or until firm. Turn off the oven and leave to cool.

■ Meanwhile, make the filling by mixing together the yogurt and strawberries in a bowl. Set aside.

■ Assemble the 'sandwiches' by placing a meringue disc on a serving plate. Top with the yogurt/strawberry mixture and top that with another meringue disc. Repeat with the remaining meringues and the yogurt mixture. Lightly dust with cocoa and icing sugar, if desired, and serve garnished with mint leaves.

**BONUS POINT**
The meringue discs can be prepared up to a day in advance and kept in an air-tight container.

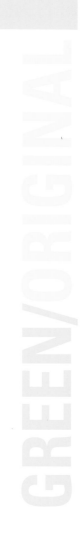

GREEN/ORIGINAL

**serves** 4
**preparation time**
20 minutes
**cooking time**
12–15 minutes
**vegetarian**
**syns per serving**
original **6¹/₂**
green **6¹/₂**

# Raspberry 'custard' tarts

These thin and crisp filo shells are filled with orange-flavoured custard and topped with juicy raspberries to create a wonderful dessert.

Fry Light for spraying
4 large sheets fresh filo pastry
150g/5oz Quark soft cheese
100g/3½ oz low fat custard

1 tbsp finely grated orange zest
200g/7oz raspberries
icing sugar (optional)

■ Preheat the oven to 180°C/Gas 4. Spray four individual tartlet tins with Fry Light.

■ Cut each sheet of filo pastry into four squares. Spray the squares with Fry Light and line each tin with four of the squares, placed at different angles to form a pastry case. Place in the oven and bake for 12–15 minutes until lightly golden and crisp. Remove from the oven and from the tins and allow to cool on a wire rack.

■ Make the 'custard' by mixing together the Quark, custard, orange zest and half of the raspberries.

■ To serve, place the pastry cases on individual plates and spoon in the 'custard' mixture. Top each serving with the remaining raspberries and lightly dust with icing sugar, if using. Serve immediately.

**BONUS POINT**
The filo tartlets can be made a couple of days ahead and kept in an air-tight container until ready to serve.

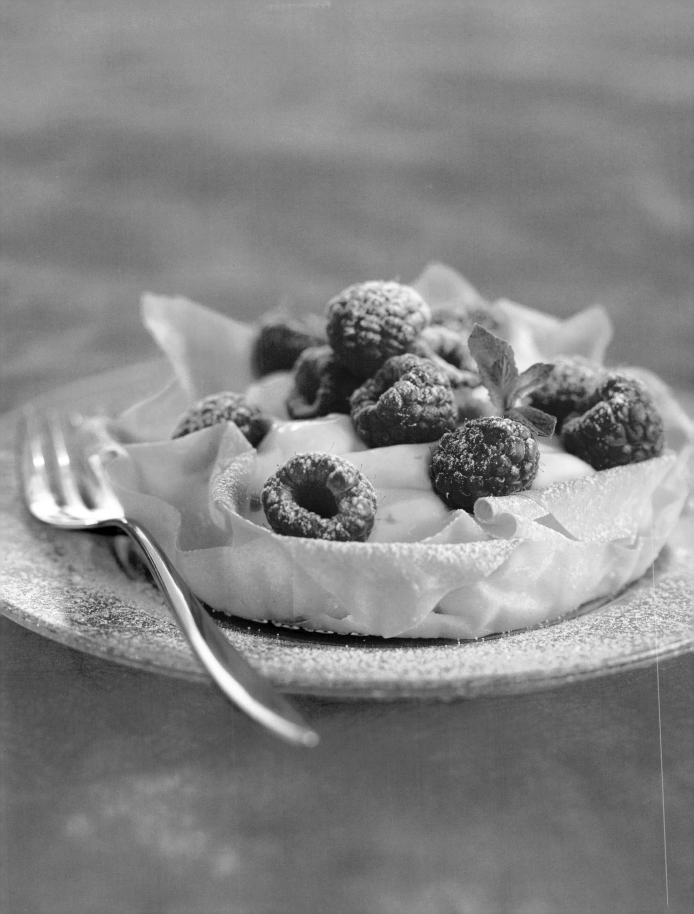

**makes** 32 squares
**preparation time**
10 minutes
**cooking time**
30–35 minutes
**vegetarian**
**syns per square**
original **4 per square**
green **4 per square**

# Orange and chocolate chip squares

Served with berries and very low fat yogurt, these delicious chocolate squares are relatively low in Syns and really easy to make.

Fry Light for spraying
350g/12oz self-raising flour
175g/6oz golden caster sugar
100g/3½ oz low fat spread
1 tbsp finely grated orange zest
1 x 200g/7oz pot Müllerlight vanilla-
  flavoured yogurt

1 egg, lightly beaten
100g/3½ oz chocolate chips or pieces
a few drops of vanilla essence

to serve:
mixed berries
very low fat natural yogurt

Preheat the oven to 180°C/Gas 4. Lightly spray a non-stick Swiss-roll tin with Fry Light.

Place the flour, sugar, low fat spread, orange zest, yogurt and egg in a food processor and blend until smooth. Fold in the chocolate chips and the vanilla and spoon the mixture into the Swiss-roll tin.

Cook in the oven for 30–35 minutes or until the mixture is set and cooked through the middle. Allow to cool before cutting into squares. The squares can be served with a selection of berries and a dollop of yogurt, if desired.

**BONUS POINT**
You can store the squares for one to two days in an air-tight container.

# Crêpes with mixed fruit

Prepare the crêpes ahead of time so you can have more time with your guests and then assemble just before serving.

**serves** 4
**preparation time**
20 minutes
**cooking time**
30–35 minutes
**vegetarian**
**syns per serving**
original **3¹/₂**
green **3¹/₂**

60g/2oz plain flour
2 large eggs, lightly beaten
200g/7oz very low fat natural
  fromage frais
a few drops of vanilla essence
150ml/¼pt skimmed milk

400g/14oz roughly chopped mixed
  fruit of your choice, e.g. bananas,
  strawberries, grapes
100g/3½oz Müllerlight vanilla-
  flavoured yogurt
Fry Light for spraying
cocoa powder

▪ Sift the flour into a mixing bowl and then add the eggs, fromage frais and vanilla essence. Whisk until smooth. Add the milk and whisk to form a smooth batter. Chill for 30 minutes.

▪ Meanwhile, make the filling by mixing together the chopped mixed fruit and yogurt and set aside.

▪ Lightly spray a small non-stick frying pan with Fry Light over a medium heat and when hot add a small ladleful of the batter, swirling to cover the base. Cook the crêpe for 1–2 minutes on each side until lightly golden at the edges and just set. Remove and stack between non-stick parchment paper. Repeat to make seven more crêpes.

▪ To serve, place two pancakes on each serving plate and top each with the mixed fruit mixture. Fold over carefully and serve immediately, dusted lightly with cocoa powder.

**BONUS POINT**
For alternative flavourings, try using other Müllerlight yogurts.

GREEN/ORIGINAL

205

**serves** 12
**preparation time**
25 minutes
**cooking time**
25–30 minutes
**vegetarian**
**syns per serving**
original **3**
green **3**

# Orange and almond drizzle cake

This rich-tasting cake, with a zesty, orange-flavoured drizzle, is relatively low in Syns and very, very tasty!

**Fry Light for spraying**
**4 large eggs**
**60g/2oz golden caster sugar**
**4 tbsp artificial sweetener**
**100g/3½ oz self-raising flour**
**1 level tsp baking powder**
**2 level tbsp ground almonds**
**1 tbsp finely grated orange zest**

**for the drizzle:**
**juice of 2 sweet oranges**
**1 tbsp arrowroot**
**4–5 tbsp artificial sweetener**
**1 tbsp finely grated orange zest**

**to serve:**
**fresh orange segments**
**very low fat natural fromage frais**
**  (optional)**

Preheat the oven to 190°C/Gas 5. Spray a 22cm/8½in diameter, loose-bottomed cake tin with Fry Light and line with non-stick baking parchment.

In a clean bowl whisk the eggs, sugar and sweetener until the mixture is thick and leaves a trail. In a separate bowl mix together the flour, baking powder and almonds and fold into the egg mixture with a metal spoon. Stir in the orange zest. Spoon this mixture into the prepared tin, place in the oven and bake for 25–30 minutes or until the cake has risen and is just firm to the touch. Leave to cool.

**BONUS POINT**
While the cake will store well for up to three days in an air-tight container, the drizzle should be made just before serving.

Meanwhile, make the drizzle by heating the orange juice with 60ml/2fl oz water in a small saucepan. Whisk in the arrowroot, sweetener and orange zest. Bring to the boil and cook for a few minutes until it thickens. Remove from the heat and leave to cool. To serve, cut the cake into 12 wedges and spoon over the orange drizzle. Serve with orange segments and fromage frais, if desired.

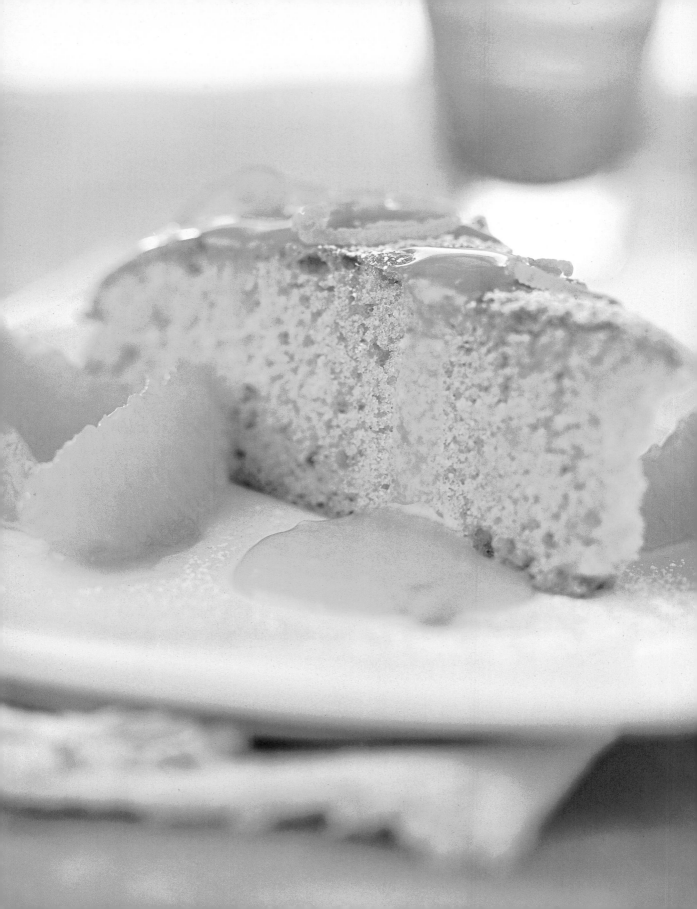

GREEN/ORIGINAL

**serves** 4
**preparation time**
10 minutes
**cooking time**
about 15 minutes
**vegetarian**
**syns per serving**
original **2**
green **2**

# Poached plums with vanilla cream

Cinnamon, star anise and orange gently flavour these juicy poached plums, which are served chilled with a cinnamon and vanilla cream.

250ml/8fl oz diluted, sugar-free
   blackcurrant squash
1 star anise
1 cinnamon stick
2–3 cloves
1 tbsp finely grated orange zest
2 cardamom pods, lightly crushed
5 tbsp artificial sweetener

450g/16oz ripe plums

for the cream:
250g/9oz very low fat natural
   fromage frais
1/2 tsp vanilla essence
1 tsp ground cinnamon
4 tbsp artificial sweetener

Pour the blackcurrant squash into a medium-sized saucepan and add the star anise, cinnamon stick, cloves, orange zest and cardamom. Place over a medium heat and bring to the boil. Simmer gently for 3–4 minutes before adding the sweetener and the plums.

Cover the pan and reduce the heat to low. Simmer gently for 8–10 minutes or until the plums are tender. Remove the plums with a slotted spoon and transfer to a serving bowl.

Bring the syrup in the pan to the boil and take off the heat. Strain into a little jug or bowl and discard the whole spices. Pour this liquid over the plums, cover and chill until ready to serve.

Meanwhile, make the cream by mixing together all the ingredients. Divide the plums and their poaching liquid between four dessert bowls and serve with the cream.

**BONUS POINT**
Try poaching small pears as an alternative, or even apricots or peaches.

# Jamaican **banana** and **rum** flambé

serves 4
**preparation time**
10 minutes
**cooking time**
5–6 minutes
**vegetarian**
**syns per serving**
original **6**
green **6**

Rum, ginger and lime are the flavours of this tropical dessert, which marry terrifically well with the grilled bananas and vanilla yogurt.

**Fry Light for spraying**
**1 level tbsp golden caster sugar**
**1 tsp ground ginger**
**4 firm bananas**
**finely grated zest and juice of 1 lime**
**3 tbsp dark rum**

**1 x 200g/7oz pot Müllerlight vanilla-**
  **flavoured yogurt**

Line a grill rack with foil and lightly spray with Fry Light. Mix together the sugar and the ground ginger and set aside.

Peel the bananas and cut each one diagonally into 3–4 pieces and place on the grill rack.

Sprinkle the sugar and ginger mixture over the banana pieces and sprinkle over the lime zest and juice.

Preheat the grill to high and place the bananas under the grill. Cook for 3–4 minutes or until golden and then transfer the bananas and any juices that have collected on the foil to a shallow serving bowl.

Place the rum in a metal ladle and carefully hold over a medium heat until warmed. Using a match, set the rum alight in the ladle and then pour the flaming rum over the bananas. Serve immediately with the vanilla yogurt.

**BONUS POINT**
If desired, you could substitute chopped pineapple for the bananas.

**GREEN/ORIGINAL**

209

serves 4
**preparation time**
20 minutes +
freezing
**vegetarian**
**syns per serving**
original **2¹/₂**
green **2¹/₂**

# Minted watermelon granita with shaved melon

Nothing compares to this home-made ice, which, if made with sweet, ripe watermelons, is a real treat, especially on a hot summer's day.

**¹/₂ small, ripe watermelon**
**1 tbsp lemon juice**
**2–3 tbsp artificial sweetener**
**1 tbsp very finely chopped mint leaves**

**to serve:**
**¹/₂ Galia or Charentais melon**

Make the granita by cutting the watermelon flesh into large chunks and discarding the seeds. Place in a blender with the lemon juice, sweetener and finely chopped mint leaves. Process until smooth and then pour into a large, shallow, freezerproof container so that the mixture is not more than 2.5cm/1in deep.

Cover and freeze for 2–3 hours until the mixture around the sides starts to form crystals. Mash the granita with a metal fork and continue to freeze for a further 2 hours, mashing the mixture every 30 minutes until the consistency is grainy and slushy. Freeze until required.

To serve, peel the Galia or Charentais melon and cut into very thin slices. Divide the granita between four glasses and top with melon slices. Serve immediately.

**BONUS POINT**
If the granita has frozen too solid, remove it from the freezer for 15–20 minutes or until you are able to scoop it with ease.

GREEN/ORIGINAL

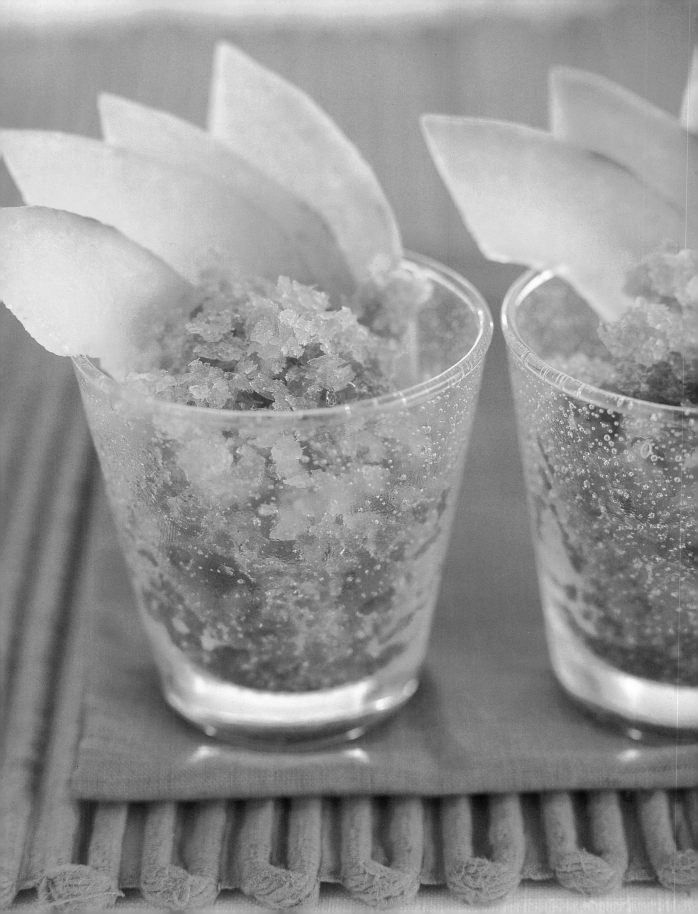

serves 4
**preparation time**
15–20 minutes +
chilling
**vegetarian**
**syns per serving**
original **3¹/₂**
green **3¹/₂**

# Rhubarb, ginger and mandarin syllabub

This delectable dessert, low in Syns, is great for entertaining as it can be prepared ahead of time and chilled until ready to serve.

600g/1lb 6oz rhubarb
60g/2oz golden caster sugar
1 tsp finely grated ginger
finely grated zest and juice of 2
   mandarins
2 seedless mandarins, peeled and
   segmented

1 x 200g/7oz pot Müllerlight
   mandarin-flavoured yogurt

to garnish:
mint leaves

Wash the rhubarb and cut into small pieces and place in a saucepan with the sugar, grated ginger and the mandarin zest and juice. Place over a medium heat, cover and cook for 12–15 minutes, stirring occasionally, until the rhubarb is tender. Remove from the heat and allow to cool. When cool, place in the fridge and chill for 3–4 hours or overnight, if time permits.

When ready to serve, divide the mandarin segments between four chilled dessert glasses or bowls and then layer the rhubarb mixture with the yogurt. Garnish with mint leaves and serve chilled.

**BONUS POINT**
When rhubarb is out of season, substitute peeled and chopped apples and pears in its place.

GREEN/ORIGINAL

## Apricot compote with spiced custard

Orange, vanilla and cardamom-scented custard makes a perfect partner for these lightly stewed apricots. For maximum effect, serve well chilled.

**serves** 4
**preparation time**
about 25 minutes
+ chilling
**vegetarian**
**syns per serving**
original **6**
green **6**

8 large, ripe apricots
200ml/7fl oz orange juice
1 large lemon
60g/2oz golden caster sugar
1 vanilla pod, split in half lengthways
3 tbsp artificial sweetener
3 tbsp finely chopped mint leaves

for the custard:
150g/5oz low fat custard
1 tbsp finely grated orange zest
$1/4$ tsp ground cinnamon
$1/4$ tsp vanilla essence
$1/4$ tsp crushed cardamom seeds

■ Wash the apricots and cut each into half, discarding the stone. Cut into quarters and place in a saucepan with the orange juice. Cut the lemon in half and squeeze over the juice and add the golden caster sugar, vanilla pod, sweetener and mint leaves.

■ Place the pan over a medium heat and bring to the boil. Cover, reduce the heat and cook gently for 8–10 minutes or until the fruit is just tender. Remove from the heat and remove the fruit with a slotted spoon to four dessert bowls. Cover and chill in the fridge.

■ Place the remaining liquid in the pan over a high heat and bring to the boil and cook for 5–6 minutes. Remove and allow to cool. When cool, chill in the fridge until ready to serve.

■ Make the custard by combining all the ingredients in a small bowl. To serve, pour the cooled syrup over the cooked apricots and top with the spiced custard.

**BONUS POINT**
For a subtle change in flavour, substitute apple juice for the orange juice.

GREEN/ORIGINAL

# Recipe Syn Values

The Syns listed for each of the recipes in this book are per portion.

## ORIGINAL DAY RECIPES

| THE BIG BREAKFAST | Page | Original | Green |
|---|---|---|---|
| Fruity French toast | 42 | 4$^1$/$_2$ | 4$^1$/$_2$ |
| Herby smoked salmon scrambled eggs | 54 | free | 2 |
| Pick-me-up breakfast hash | 56 | 3 | 11 |
| Minted summer fruit vanilla smoothie | 59 | 1$^1$/$_2$ | 1$^1$/$_2$ |

| PORTABLE LUNCHES & PICNICS | | | |
|---|---|---|---|
| Courgette, red pepper and mint frittata | 62 | 1 | 1 |
| Chilled summer gazpacho | 72 | $^1$/$_2$ | $^1$/$_2$ |
| Dill, lemon and tuna dip | 75 | free | 5 |
| Stuffed cabbage leaves | 76 | free | 2 |
| Tuna, cucumber and baby gem salad | 78 | $^1$/$_2$ | 5$^1$/$_2$ |
| Chicken and tarragon terrine with rustic tomato sauce | 80 | 1$^1$/$_2$ | 9$^1$/$_2$ |

| LIGHT SALAD LUNCHES | | | |
|---|---|---|---|
| Mixed grilled pepper and basil salad | 84 | $^1$/$_2$ | $^1$/$_2$ |
| Feta, watermelon and olive salad | 90 | 3$^1$/$_2$ | 3$^1$/$_2$ |
| North African carrot and coriander salad | 91 | $^1$/$_2$ | $^1$/$_2$ |
| Prawn, mango and herb salad | 96 | $^1$/$_2$ | 9$^1$/$_2$ |
| Creamy Caesar's salad with croûtons | 98 | 3 | 4$^1$/$_2$ |
| Fruity chicken salad with a creamy tarragon and mustard dressing | 100 | $^1$/$_2$ | 8 |
| Warm spiced chicken and spinach salad | 102 | free | 10$^1$/$_2$ |
| Spicy Thai-style beef salad | 103 | free | 8 |

| MIDWEEK FAMILY SUPPERS | | | |
|---|---|---|---|
| Provençal pan-cooked chicken | 116 | $^1$/$_2$ | 10 |
| Herb and garlic chicken Kievs | 118 | 2 | 9$^1$/$_2$ |
| Pork and apple stew with swede mash | 119 | 3$^1$/$_2$ | 10$^1$/$_2$ |
| Pork and mushroom stroganoff | 120 | free | 10 |
| Luxury chilli con carne | 121 | 5$^1$/$_2$ | 16$^1$/$_2$ |
| Lemon and rosemary lamb skewers with aubergine purée | 122 | free | 6 |
| Oriental beef and mixed pepper stir-fry | 124 | free | 9 |

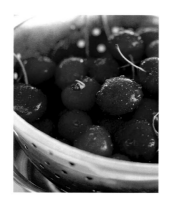
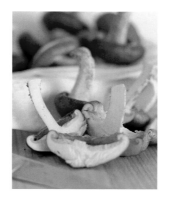
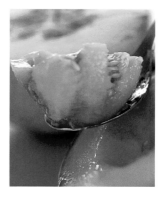

## TEA-TIME TREATS

| TEA-TIME TREATS | Page | Original | Green |
|---|---|---|---|
| Vegetable samosas with mint chutney | 128 | 3 | 3 |
| Toasted triple decker | 131 | 3 | 3 |
| Sardinian-style vegetable pizza | 134 | 4 | 4 |
| Grilled pepper and olive bruschetta | 136 | 6$\frac{1}{2}$ | 6$\frac{1}{2}$ |
| Long Island seafood skewers with a basil and tomato dip | 138 | 1 | 8 |
| Spicy glazed chicken wings | 140 | 2 | 10 |
| Bangers and champ | 141 | 5$\frac{1}{2}$ | 9 |
| Blueberry muffins | 142 | 3 | 3 |
| Strawberry and sultana scones | 144 | 3 | 3 |
| Mini citrus fruit bakewells | 145 | 2$\frac{1}{2}$ | 2$\frac{1}{2}$ |
| Moist banana bread | 146 | 4$\frac{1}{2}$ | 4$\frac{1}{2}$ |
| Gingerbread squares | 147 | 3$\frac{1}{2}$ | 3$\frac{1}{2}$ |
| White and dark chocolate chip cookies | 148 | 2$\frac{1}{2}$ | 2$\frac{1}{2}$ |

## SUNDAY BRUNCHES & ROAST LUNCHES

| SUNDAY BRUNCHES & ROAST LUNCHES | Page | Original | Green |
|---|---|---|---|
| Eggs benedict | 152 | 6$\frac{1}{2}$ | 9$\frac{1}{2}$ |
| Apple, ginger and cinnamon milkshake | 155 | 3$\frac{1}{2}$ | 3$\frac{1}{2}$ |
| Pancake and fruit stack | 156 | 7 | 7 |
| Cauliflower, chive and cheese gratin | 159 | 5 | 5 |
| Creamy rocket and mustard mash | 160 | $\frac{1}{2}$ | $\frac{1}{2}$ |
| Honey and mustard roast salmon with roasted ratatouille | 164 | $\frac{1}{2}$ | 15$\frac{1}{2}$ |
| Roasted spiced pesto chicken | 166 | free | 7$\frac{1}{2}$ |
| Citrus and garlic roasted poussins | 167 | free | 10$\frac{1}{2}$ |
| Mediterranean lamb and carrot stew | 168 | 2 | 13$\frac{1}{2}$ |
| Sausage roast with celeriac mash | 169 | 4$\frac{1}{2}$ | 10$\frac{1}{2}$ |
| Peppered roast beef with roasted root vegetables | 170 | | |
|     If serving 6 | | $\frac{1}{2}$ | 15$\frac{1}{2}$ |
|     If serving 8 | | $\frac{1}{2}$ | 11$\frac{1}{2}$ |

## EASY, EXOTIC & ELEGANT ENTERTAINING

## DESSERTS TO DIE FOR

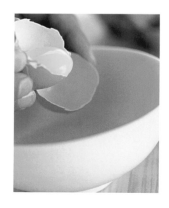
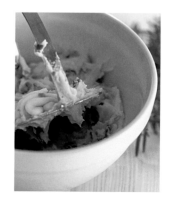
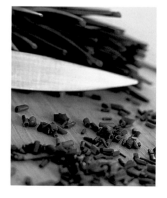

# GREEN DAY RECIPES

| THE BIG BREAKFAST | Page | Original | Green |
|---|---|---|---|
| Fruity French toast | 42 | 4¹/₂ | 4¹/₂ |
| Root vegetable rostis | 44 | 7 | free |
| Breakfast corn slice | 45 | 1¹/₂ | free |
| Potato and spring onion pancakes | 46 | 8 | free |
| Egg and tomato bakes with parsnip chips | 48 | | |
| Egg and tomato bakes | | free | free |
| Parsnip chips | | 5¹/₂ | free |
| Celeriac chips | | free | free |
| Club-style bean burger breakfast | 55 | 11¹/₂ | 6 |
| Smoked salmon kedgeree | 58 | 6¹/₂ | 3¹/₂ |
| Minted summer fruit vanilla smoothie | 59 | 1¹/₂ | 1¹/₂ |

| PORTABLE LUNCHES & PICNICS | | | |
|---|---|---|---|
| Courgette, red pepper and mint frittata | 62 | 1 | 1 |
| West coast sunshine pasta salad | 64 | 12 | ¹/₂ |
| Herby tabbouleh salad | 65 | 12 | ¹/₂ |
| Roasted 'al fresco' vegetable couscous | 66 | 9 | free |
| Fragrant stuffed vine leaves | 69 | 4¹/₂ | free |
| Spicy chickpea balls with yogurt relish | 70 | 6 | ¹/₂ |
| Jewelled vegetable picnic paella | 71 | 18¹/₂ | free |
| Chilled summer gazpacho | 72 | ¹/₂ | ¹/₂ |
| Vichyssoise | 74 | 2 | ¹/₂ |
| Spicy Mexican roll | 79 | 14 | 8 |

| LIGHT SALAD LUNCHES | | | |
|---|---|---|---|
| Mixed grilled pepper and basil salad | 84 | ¹/₂ | ¹/₂ |
| Creamy Quorn, vegetable and pasta salad | 86 | 9 | free |
| Ultimate celery, apple and potato salad | 87 | 7 | 1¹/₂ |
| Farfalle and mixed bean salad | 88 | 8 | free |
| Feta, watermelon and olive salad | 90 | 3¹/₂ | 3¹/₂ |
| North African carrot and coriander salad | 91 | ¹/₂ | ¹/₂ |
| Harlequin rice salad | 92 | 4¹/₂ | free |
| Puy lentil salad | 94 | 3¹/₂ | free |
| Chilled Russian salad | 95 | 3 | 1¹/₂ |
| French-style bean and tuna salad | 99 | 7 | 5 |

| MIDWEEK FAMILY SUPPERS | Page | Original | Green |
|---|---|---|---|
| Fragrant carrot, pea and tomato pilaff | 106 | 18½ | free |
| Spinach and courgette cannelloni | 108 | 6½ | ½ |
| Special macaroni cheese | 109 | 24 | 6½ |
| Roasted vegetable lasagne | 110 | 9 | 3 |
| Spaghetti Bolognese | 112 | 23 | ½ |
| Piquant vegetable cottage pie | 114 | 9 | 1 |
| Fish and 'chips' with 'tartar' sauce | 115 | 10 | 8 |
| Italian-style spaghetti and meatballs | 125 | 15 | 11½ |

| TEA-TIME TREATS | | | |
|---|---|---|---|
| Vegetable samosas with mint chutney | 128 | 3 | 3 |
| Crispy stuffed potato skins | 130 | 8 | free |
| Toasted triple decker | 131 | 3 | 3 |
| Tex-mex chilli burritos | 132 | 6 | 3½ |
| Pea and tomato tortilla | 133 | 2 | free |
| Sardinian-style vegetable pizza | 134 | 4 | 4 |
| Grilled pepper and olive bruschetta | 136 | 6½ | 6½ |
| Irish potato cakes | 137 | 5½ | free |
| Blueberry muffins | 142 | 3 | 3 |
| Strawberry and sultana scones | 144 | 3 | 3 |
| Mini citrus fruit bakewells | 145 | 2½ | 2½ |
| Moist banana bread | 146 | 4½ | 4½ |
| Gingerbread squares | 147 | 3½ | 3½ |
| White and dark chocolate chip cookies | 148 | 2½ | 2½ |

| SUNDAY BRUNCHES & ROAST LUNCHES | | | |
|---|---|---|---|
| Sweet potato wedges with chilli 'mayo' | 154 | 6 | free |
| Apple, ginger and cinnamon milkshake | 155 | 3½ | 3½ |
| Pancake and fruit stack | 156 | 7 | 7 |
| Chunky root vegetable hot pot | 158 | 7 | free |
| Cauliflower, chive and cheese gratin | 159 | 5 | 5 |
| Creamy rocket and mustard mash | 160 | ½ | ½ |
| Chilli and coriander mash | 160 | 8 | free |
| Vegetable shepherd's pie | 162 | 9 | 3½ |
| Spanish-style oven-baked vegetable rice | 163 | 9½ | free |

| EASY, EXOTIC & ELEGANT ENTERTAINING | | | |
|---|---|---|---|
| Vegetable biryani | 174 | 18 | ½ |
| Minted asparagus risotto | 177 | 12 | ½ |
| Middle Eastern vegetable casserole with couscous | 188 | 11 | ½ |

## DESSERTS TO DIE FOR

# FREE FOOD RECIPES

## THE BIG BREAKFAST

## PORTABLE LUNCHES & PICNICS

## MIDWEEK FAMILY SUPPERS

## SUNDAY BRUNCHES & ROAST LUNCHES

## EASY, EXOTIC & ELEGANT ENTERTAINING

**S =** weight loss boost
**SS =** extra weight loss boost
**F =** extra fibre
**FF =** extra rich fibre
**H =** healthy
**HH =** vital to health

# Free Foods selection

**We have listed many of our Free Foods here. For the full list, you will need to become a Slimming World member.**

■ Foods marked with an S symbol will give your weight loss a boost. Choosing foods marked with an SS symbol will give your weight loss an even bigger boost.

■ Foods marked with an F will give you extra fibre and those marked with FF will give you an even richer helping of fibre.

■ Foods marked H will keep you healthy and those marked HH are vital to your health and need to be included in your diet every day.

## GREEN CHOICE FREE FOODS

**All vegetables are classed as a Free Food when on a Green day.**

| | | | |
|---|---|---|---|
| Potatoes | | | HH |
| Rice | | | H |
| Dried pasta | | | H |
| Buckwheat | | | H |
| Couscous | | | H |
| Baked beans | F | SS | H |
| Chick peas | F | | H |
| Red kidney beans | FF | S | H |
| Soya beans | FF | | H |
| Lentils | F | S | H |
| Peas | F | SS | H |
| Quorn | F | SS | H |

**The following fruits can be eaten freely as long as they are fresh or frozen varieties.**

| | | |
|---|---|---|
| Apples | S | HH |
| Bananas | | HH |
| Grapefruit | SS | HH |
| Oranges | S | HH |
| Peaches | | S |
| HH | | |
| Pineapple | S | HH |
| Strawberries | SS | HH |
| | | |
| Eggs | | |
| Tofu | | |
| Very low fat natural yogurt | | H |

## ORIGINAL CHOICE FREE FOODS

**Not all vegetables are Free Foods on the Original Choice. Choose freely from the following list:**

| | | | |
|---|---|---|---|
| Artichokes | F | S | HH |
| Asparagus | | S | HH |
| Aubergine | | S | HH |
| Beans – French, runner | F | S | HH |
| Beetroot | | S | HH |
| Broccoli | F | S | HH |
| Brussels sprouts | F | S | HH |
| Cabbage | | S | HH |
| Carrots | | S | HH |
| Cauliflower | | S | HH |
| Courgettes | | S | HH |
| Leeks | | S | HH |
| Mushrooms | | S | HH |
| Onions | | S | HH |
| Spinach | | S | HH |
| Squash | | S | HH |
| Swede | | S | HH |
| Sweetcorn - baby whole | | S | HH |
| Quorn | F | SS | H |

**The following fruits can be eaten freely as long as they are fresh or frozen varieties.**

| | | |
|---|---|---|
| Apples | S | HH |
| Bananas | | HH |
| Oranges | S | HH |
| Grapes | | HH |
| Pineapple | S | HH |
| Strawberries | SS | HH |

**Dairy**

| | | |
|---|---|---|
| Eggs | | |
| Very low fat natural yogurt | | H |
| Very low fat natural fromage frais | | H |

**Poultry**

| | | |
|---|---|---|
| Chicken, no fat or skin | S | H |
| Turkey, no fat or skin | S | H |

**Meat**

| |
|---|
| Bacon |
| Beef |

## ORIGINAL CHOICE FREE FOODS (continued)

| | | | | | |
|---|---|---|---|---|---|
| Ham | | | Pilchards | | H |
| Lamb | | | Plaice | SS | H |
| Pork | | | Salmon (fresh, canned and smoked) | | H |
| **Fish** | | | Sole | SS | H |
| Cod | SS | H | | | |
| Haddock | SS | H | **Shellfish** | | |
| Kippers | | H | Crab | | H |
| Mackerel (not smoked) | | H | Prawns | S | H |

# Syns selection

■ Listed below are a selection of Syn values for foods that you can enjoy every day. The values apply to both Green and Original days.

## ALCOHOL
25ml/1fl oz measure of
   any spirit 2¹/₂
150ml/¹/₄ pt glass of wine 5
300ml/¹/₂ pt lager/beer 5
300ml/¹/₂ pt cider 5

## BISCUITS AND BARS Each
Cheese thin 1
Chocolate finger 1¹/₂
Custard cream 3
Digestive 4
Go Ahead Crispy Fruit
   Slices 3
Jaffa cake/ginger nut 2¹/₂
Jammie dodger 4
Rich tea/marie 2
Shortcake 2¹/₂
Special K Cereal Bar 4¹/₂

## CAKES Per cake, average
Chocolate mini roll 5¹/₂
McVitie's Golden Syrup
   Cake Bar 6¹/₂
Mr Kipling Angel/Lemon/
   Chocolate Slices 6¹/₂
Mr Kipling Mini Battenburg 7
Toffee Crisp Biscuit Bar 6¹/₂

## CHOCOLATE AND SWEETS
*Per standard bar/tube/bag unless stated*

Flake 9
Fudge/Curly Wurly 6¹/₂
Fun-size bars 5
Maltesers 9
Milky Bar 3¹/₂
Milky Way 6
Penguin bar 7
Polo mints 7
Two-finger Kit Kat 5¹/₂

## CRISPS Per standard bag
French Fries/Golden
   Lights 4¹/₂
Quavers 5
Snack-a-Jacks 7
Standard potato crisps,
   per 30g/1oz 7¹/₂
Thai Bites 4¹/₂
Wotsits 5¹/₂

## DESSERTS Per pot
Müllerlight Fruit Halo 4¹/₂
Müllerlight Mousse 7¹/₂
Müllerice, 99% Fat Free 6
Nestlé Aero Twist Mousse 7

If you wish to enjoy some of the delicious dessert recipes on pages 192–213, check the Syn values on the recipe page and count this into your daily allowance.

## ICE CREAMS/LOLLIES
60g/2oz scoop low fat
   ice cream 4
Fab Ice Lolly 4
Milky Way Ice Cream Bar 5¹/₂
Mini Cornetto/Calippo 3
Solero Ice 4
Strawberry Split Ice 6¹/₂

## NUTS Per 30g/1oz
Brazil nuts, shelled 9¹/₂
Cashew nuts, shelled 8
Peanuts/almonds, fresh/
   roasted 8¹/₂
Walnuts, shelled 9¹/₂

## SAUCES AND SPREADS
Custard made with
   skimmed milk:
   2 level tbsp 1
Gravy made with no fat:
   4 level tbsp 1
Margarine/spread, low
   fat variety: 30g/1oz 5¹/₂
Mayonnaise,
   reduced calorie:
   1 level tbsp 2¹/₂
Oil, any variety:
   1 level tbsp 6

index

ACKNOWLEDGMENTS
The publishers wish to thank the
following companies for supplying the
photographs that appear on the
following pages:
Iconica: page 29
Photonica: pages 19, 20, 22, 26, 27, 28
Getty Images: page 25